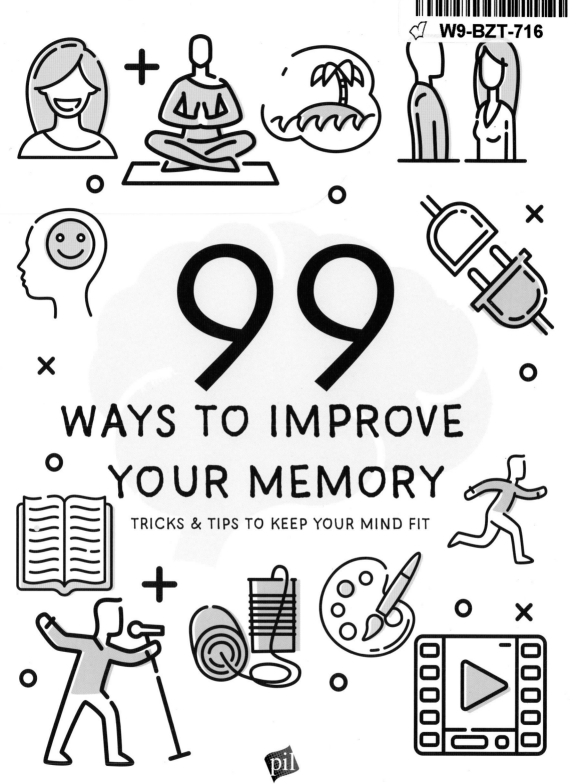

99

WAYS TO IMPROVE

YOUR MEMORY

TRICKS & TIPS TO KEEP YOUR MIND FIT

pil

Publications International, Ltd.

WHAT'S IN A BRAIN?

Research in humans strongly indicates that stimulating the brain in a variety of ways throughout life can help to protect cognitive function. It also appears to provide a kind of mental reserve that helps delay signs of normal brain aging as well as loss of cognitive function related to Alzheimer's disease and other types of dementia.

In the pages ahead, you'll discover 99 ways to improve your memory. These ideas range from the obvious—like learning a new language, an instrument, or mnemonic devices—to the nontraditional, such as karaoke or camping. You'll find helpful diet and exercise advice as well as ideas for a better night's sleep.

But first, let's talk about your brain—and how memory actually works.

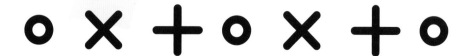

HONING YOUR MEMORY

Have you ever walked out of a mall and completely forgotten where you parked your car? If it happened to you when you were 20 years old, you probably didn't think anything of it. Once you're in your fifties and sixties, however, you may begin to wonder if such memory gaps are simply due to aging—or something worse.

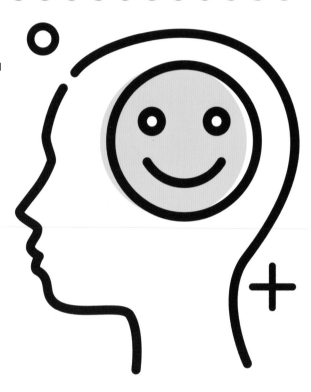

But no matter your age, occasionally forgetting where you parked your car or where you left personal items is often completely normal. It's known as "everyday forgetting," and it's so common because it involves things we do every day and usually don't spend much time paying attention to. And that lack of attention is the very reason these instances of everyday forgetting occur.

Of course, as you get older, you're more likely to think—and worry—about memory problems. And the more you worry about them, the more likely you are to notice each and every slip. Odds are you forgot quite a few things when you were in your teens and twenties, but you never paid much attention to those lapses, and you certainly didn't worry about them. The fact is, the more you expect to have

memory problems, the more you'll notice them.

The best way to stop this vicious circle is to focus on remembering instead of forgetting. Rather than expending mental energy fretting about every little memory slip, you need to pay more attention to the act of remembering. Once you begin to do this, you'll be amazed at how much better your memory will be.

Remember How Memory Works

Your baby's first cry ... the taste of your grandmother's molasses cookies ... the scent of an ocean breeze. These are memories that make up the ongoing experience of your life. They're what make you feel comfortable with familiar people and surroundings, tie your past with your present, and provide a framework for the future. In a profound way, it is our collective set of memories—our "memory" as a whole—that makes us who we are.

Most people talk about memory as if it were a thing they have, like bad eyes or a good head of hair. But your memory doesn't exist in the way a part of your body exists—it's not a "thing" you can touch. It's a concept that refers to the process of remembering. In the past, many experts were fond of describing memory as a sort of tiny filing cabinet full of individual memory folders in which information is stored away. Others likened memory to a neural supercomputer wedged under the human scalp. But today, experts believe that memory is far more complex and elusive than that—and that it is located not in one particular place in the brain but is instead a brain-wide process.

Do you remember what you had for breakfast this morning? If the image of a big plate of fried eggs and bacon popped into your mind, you didn't dredge it up from some out-of-the-way neural alleyway. Instead, that memory was the result of an incredibly complex constructive power—one that each of us possesses—that reassembled disparate memory impressions from a web-like pattern of cells scattered throughout the brain. Your "memory" is really made up of a group of systems that each plays a different role in creating, storing, and recalling your memories. When the brain processes information normally, all of these different systems work together perfectly to provide cohesive thought.

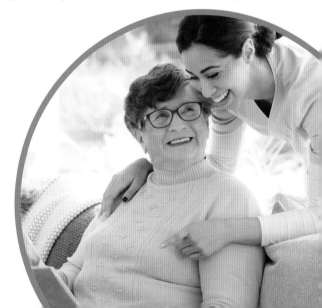

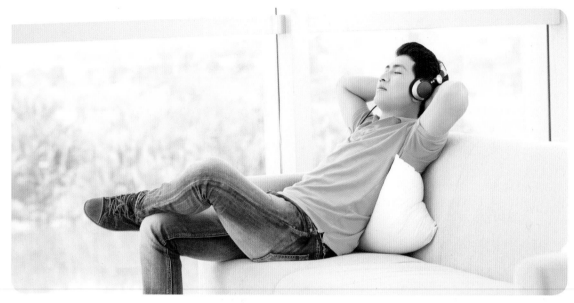

What seems to be a single memory is actually a complex construction. If you think of an object—say, a pen—your brain retrieves the object's name, its shape, its function, perhaps even the sound when it scratches across the page. Each part of the memory of what a "pen" is comes from a different region of the brain. The entire image of "pen" is actively reconstructed by the brain from many different areas. Neurologists are only beginning to understand how the parts are reassembled into a coherent whole.

If you're riding a bike, the memory of how to operate the bike comes from one set of brain cells; the memory of how to get from here to the end of the block comes from another; the memory of biking safety rules from another; and that nervous feeling you get when a car veers dangerously close, from still another. Yet you're never aware that these are separate mental experiences nor that they're coming from all different parts of your brain, because they all work together so well. In fact, experts tell us there is no firm distinction between how you remember and how you think.

This doesn't mean that scientists have figured out exactly how the system works. They still don't fully understand exactly how you remember or what occurs during recall. The search for how the brain organizes memories and where those memories are acquired and stored has been a never-ending quest among brain researchers for decades. Still, there is enough information to make some educated guesses. The process of memory begins with encoding, then proceeds to storage, and eventually moves to retrieval.

Encoding

Encoding is the first step in creating a memory. It's a biological phenomenon, rooted in the senses, that begins with perception. Consider, for example, the memory of the first person you ever fell in love with. When you met that person, your visual system likely registered physical features, such as the color of their eyes and hair. Your auditory system may have picked up the sound of their laugh. You probably noticed the scent of their perfume or cologne. You may even have felt the touch of their hand. Each of these separate sensations traveled to the part of your brain called the hippocampus, which integrated these perceptions as they were occurring into one single experience—your experience of that specific person. Experts believe that the hippocampus, along with the frontal cortex, is responsible for analyzing these various sensory inputs and deciding if they're worth remembering. If they are, they may become part of your long-term memory. As indicated earlier, these various bits of information are then stored in different parts of the brain. How these bits and pieces are later identified and retrieved to form a cohesive memory, however, is not yet known.

Although a memory begins with perception, it is encoded and stored by nerve cells using the language of electricity and chemicals. The connections between nerve cells in the brain aren't set in concrete—they change all the time. Brain cells work together in a network, organizing themselves into groups that specialize in different kinds of information processing. As one brain cell sends signals to another, the synapse between the two gets stronger. The more signals sent between them, the stronger the connection grows. Thus, with each new experience, your brain slightly rewires its physical structure. In fact, how you use your brain helps determine how your brain is organized. It is this plasticity that can help your brain rewire itself if it is ever damaged.

As you learn and experience the world and changes occur at the synapses and dendrites, more connections in your brain are created. The brain organizes and reorganizes itself in response to your experiences, forming memories triggered by the effects of outside input prompted by experience, education, or training.

These changes are reinforced with use, so that as you learn and practice new information, intricate circuits of knowledge and memory are built in the brain. If you play a piece of music over and over, for example, the repeated firing of certain cells in a certain order in your brain makes it easier to repeat this firing later on. The result: You get better at playing the music. You can play it faster, with fewer mistakes. Practice it long enough and you will play it perfectly. Yet if you stop practicing for several weeks and then try to play the piece, you may notice that the result is no longer perfect. Your brain has already begun to forget what you once knew so well.

To properly encode a memory, you must first be paying attention. Since you cannot pay attention to everything all the time, most of what you encounter every day is simply filtered out, and only a few stimuli pass into your conscious awareness. If you remembered every single thing that you noticed, your memory would be full before you even left the house in the morning. What scientists aren't sure about is whether stimuli are screened out during the sensory input stage or only after the brain processes its significance. What we do know is that how you pay attention to information may be the most important factor in how much of it you actually remember.

Easier Encoding

If you want to remember a word, thinking about how it sounds or its meaning will help. Likewise, if you use visual imagery to help memorize something — such as meeting a person named Mr. Bell and thinking of a bell when you shake hands — you're more likely to remember it. Some experts believe that using imagery helps you remember because it provides a second kind of memory encoding, and two codes are better than one.

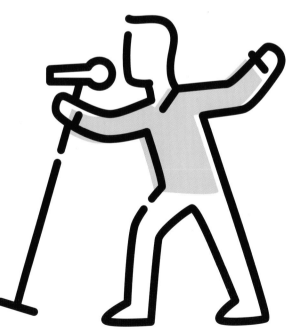

Memory Storage

Once a memory is created, it must be stored (no matter how briefly). Many experts think there are three ways we store memories: first in the sensory stage; then in short-term memory; and ultimately, for some memories, in long-term memory. Because there is no need for us to maintain everything in our brain, the different stages of human memory function as a sort of filter that helps to protect us from the flood of information that we're confronted with on a daily basis.

The creation of a memory begins with its perception: The registration of information during perception occurs in the brief sensory stage that usually lasts only a fraction of a second. It's your sensory memory that allows a perception such as a visual pattern, a sound, or a touch to linger for a brief moment after the stimulation is over.

After that first flicker, the sensation is stored in short-term memory. Short-term memory has a fairly limited

capacity; it can hold about seven items for no more than 20 or 30 seconds at a time. You may be able to increase this capacity somewhat by using various memory strategies. For example, a 10-digit number such as 8005840392 may be too much for your short-term memory to hold. But divided into chunks, as in a telephone number, 800-584-0392 may actually stay in your short-term memory long enough for you to dial the telephone. Likewise, by repeating the number to yourself, you can keep resetting the short-term memory clock.

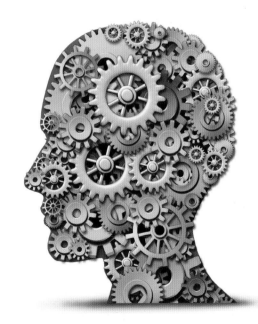

Important information is gradually transferred from short-term memory into long-term memory. The more that you repeat or use the information, the more likely it is to eventually end up in long-term memory, or be "retained." (That's why studying helps people to perform better on tests.) Unlike sensory and short-term memory, which are limited and decay rapidly, long-term memory can store unlimited amounts of information indefinitely.

People tend to more easily store material on subjects they already know, since the information has more meaning to them and can be mentally connected to related information that is already stored in their long-term memory. That's why someone who has an average memory may be able to remember a greater depth of information about one particular subject. Most people think of long-term memory when they think of "memory" itself—but most experts believe information must first pass through sensory and short-term memory before it can be stored as a long-term memory.

Types of Remembering

Psychologists have identified four types of remembering.

Recall: This is what you most often think of as "remembering"—the active, unaided remembering of something from the past.

Recollection: This is the reconstruction of events or facts on the basis of partial cues, which serve as reminders.

Recognition: This is the ability to correctly identify previously encountered stimuli—such as when you see your old teacher's face across the room and recognize who she is.

Relearning: This type of remembering is a testament to the power of the memory itself; material that's familiar to you is often easier to learn a second time.

Memory Retrieval

When you want to remember something, you retrieve the information on an unconscious level, bringing it into your conscious mind at will. While most people think they have either a "bad" or a "good" memory, in fact, most people are fairly good at remembering some types of things and not so good at remembering others. If you do have trouble remembering something—assuming you don't have a physical disease—it's usually not the fault of your entire memory system but an inefficient component of one part of your memory system.

Let's look at how you remember where you put your eyeglasses. When you go to bed at night, you must register where you place your eyeglasses: You must pay attention while you set them on your bedside table.

You must be aware of where you are putting them, or you won't be able to remember their location the following morning. Next, this information is retained, ready to be retrieved at a later time. If the system is working properly, when you wake up in the morning you will remember exactly where you left your eyeglasses.

If you've forgotten where they are, you may not have registered clearly where you put them. Or you may not have retained what you registered. Or you may not be able to retrieve the memory accurately. Therefore, if you want to stop forgetting where you left your eyeglasses, you will have to work on making sure that all three stages of the remembering process are working properly.

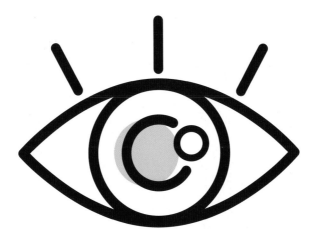

If you've forgotten something, it may be because you didn't encode it very effectively, because you were distracted while encoding should have taken place, or because you're having trouble retrieving it. If you've "forgotten" where you put your eyeglasses, you may not have really forgotten at all—instead, the location may never have gotten into your memory in the first place.

Distractions that occur while you're trying to remember something can really get in the way of encoding memories. If you're trying to read a business report in the middle of a busy airport, you may think you're remembering what you read, but you may not have effectively saved it in your memory.

Finally, you may forget because you're simply having trouble retrieving the memory. If you've ever tried to remember something one time and couldn't, but then later you remember that same item, it could be that there was a mismatch between retrieval cues and the encoding of the information you were searching for.

You'll be better able to remember something if you use a "retrieval cue" that occurred when you first formed a memory. If you memorized a poem outdoors when birds were singing, then playing birdsong might help you recall the poem. This is why vivid memories will recur strongly when you experience a sensation that accompanied the original event. It's why, for example, the sound of a car backfiring may trigger an unpleasant memory of a battlefield experience for someone who was previously in a war zone.

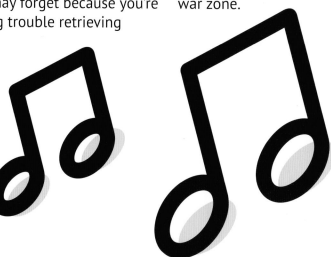

Expand Your Mind's Horizons

As long as you stay active, interested in life, and engaged in the world around you, your memory and other cognitive abilities don't have to deteriorate as you grow older. Research shows that enriching your surroundings, your daily experiences, and your life as a whole can pay off in a sharper, more resilient mind.

For example, animal studies have found that rats living in cages with plenty of exciting toys and lots of stimulation have larger, healthier brain cells and a larger outer brain layer. Deprived rats living in barren cages, on the other hand, have smaller brains.

Research in humans strongly indicates that stimulating the brain in a variety of ways throughout life can help to protect cognitive function. It also appears to provide a kind of mental reserve that helps delay signs of normal brain aging as well as loss of cognitive function.

What can you do to enrich your brain's environment? Turn the page and discover 99 ways to improve your memory—and your life!

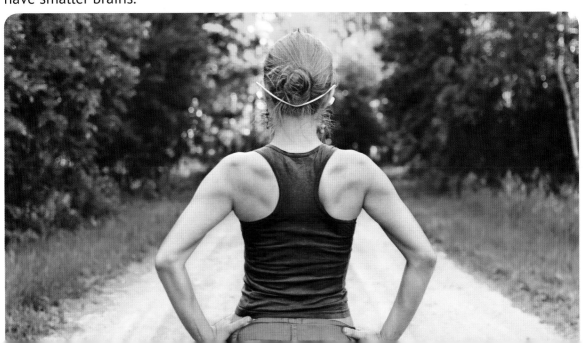

1 Take a Hike

Literature and poetry are filled with odes to nature. From Henry David Thoreau's reflective *Walden* to Robert Frost's famous wanderings through the woods, authors have sung the praises of the great outdoors for centuries. And it turns out there may be a reason that so many writers have found their muse in nature: being outdoors has been shown to increase creativity and relieve mental fatigue and burnout. It's a natural cure for writer's block!

Simply being outdoors can reduce stress and increase happiness, with studies showing that the mere observation of natural surroundings—even looking out a window—can lower heart rate. But for the biggest brain benefit, scientists recommend adding exercise, such as a hike through the woods. With its combination of fresh air and heart-pumping physical activity, a hike may not only reduce stress and boost your mood, but it could have memory-improving benefits, as well.

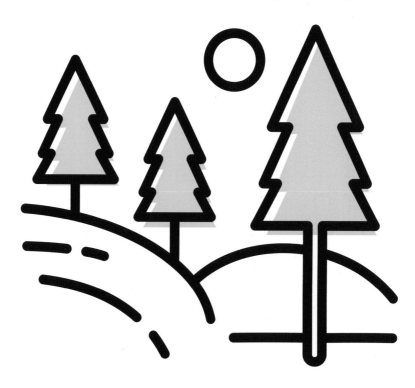

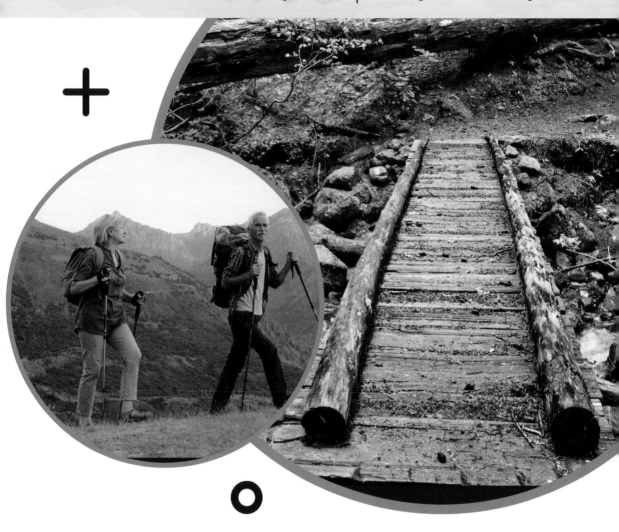

Regular exercise has been shown to increase the size of the hippocampus—the area of the brain responsible for memory—and may also boost other areas of the brain that control thinking and learning. Studies show that 120 minutes of moderate exercise a week can have a positive effect, so just a couple hour-long hikes (or several shorter ones) may be beneficial. This combination of exercise and natural surroundings literally changes the activity of the brain, making it easier to recall information, pay attention, and even solve puzzles.

So put down the smartphone, turn off the television, and head into nature—your brain will thank you for it!

2 Go Canoeing or Kayaking

The physical and psychological benefits of being in nature are undeniable. The Japanese even developed a practice known as "Shinrin-yoku," or "forest bathing," which is a key element in Japanese preventive medicine. Very simply, those who practice Shinrin-yoku regularly take time to commune with nature, which has been proven to lower blood pressure, reduce anxiety, increase focus, improve sleep, and even boost the immune system.

There is even evidence that "bathing" in nature exposes us to airborne microbes and chemicals that we would not otherwise encounter, and the exposure to this biodiversity is extremely beneficial. The unique microbes found in nature can strengthen immune function, influence mood, and lower stress hormones.

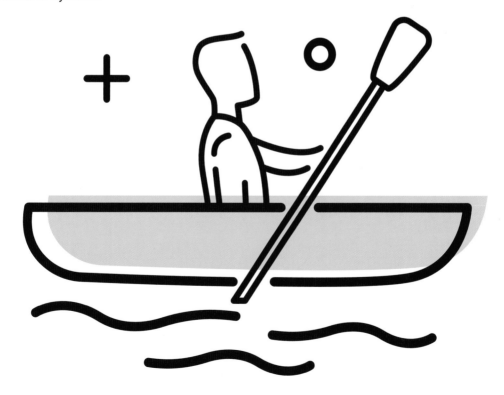

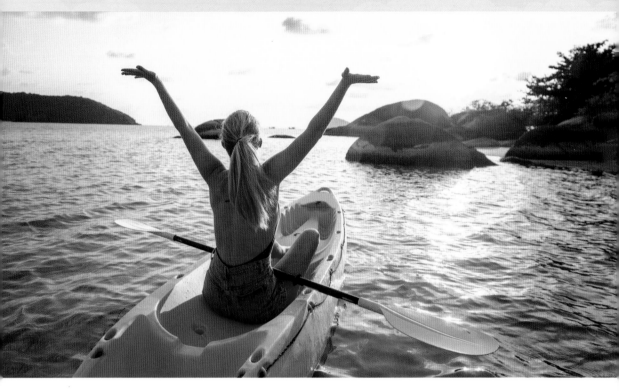

But not everyone is able to hike the rough terrain of a forest trail or climb over rocks. Canoeing and kayaking provide a low-impact way to absorb all the benefits that nature has to offer, without any impact to the knees or hips. But don't assume it's not a good workout: paddling a canoe or kayak can be as calm as a float down a quiet stream, or as strenuous as a ride through the rapids—it's up to you!

Either way, this water-logged workout has been shown to protect and change the brain in ways that improve memory and learning, as well as increase levels of dopamine, serotonin, and norepinephrine, which help to increase focus. A paddle down a lazy river may be all you need to keep your heart—and head—happy.

3 Paint Your Home New Colors

A fresh coat of paint is an easy and inexpensive way to spruce up any room in your house. Different colors can make a room look larger or smaller, provide an instant mood boost, promote restfulness, and induce calm. Take the color green, for instance—this hue is reminiscent of the grass and trees in nature, which is known to have stress-relieving properties of its own. Viewing the color green can have the same calming effects, which, in turn, helps to increase concentration and focus. This makes it an excellent color for an office environment.

And the effectiveness of this color isn't just anecdotal; studies have shown that people who work in offices with green walls report more job satisfaction, and students who gaze at green before taking a test are better able to concentrate. It may seem unlikely that a color could have such an effect, but in its purest form, color is energy. Colors are part of the electromagnetic spectrum, and each has its own magnetic frequency, which, amazingly, can create biochemical responses in our brains.

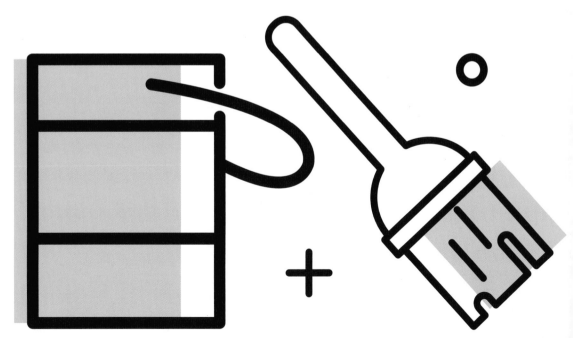

Certain colors can even improve memory and the ability to concentrate. One study focused on the colors red and blue, with participants performing cognitive tasks while looking at the colors. The study concluded that the color red boosted memory retention by as much as 31 percent.

Other colors associated with improved memory include orange, yellow, and mauve. So maybe it's time to give your brain a boost and add some colorful accents to those neutral walls.

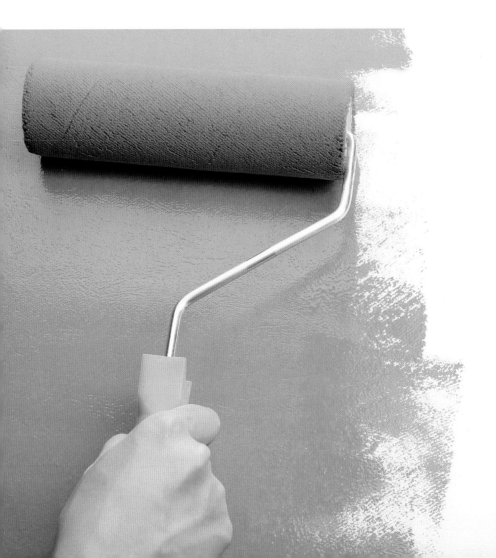

4 Travel Somewhere New

Every year, Americans leave millions of unused vacation days on the table, with surveys showing that a majority of U.S. adults haven't traveled at all in the last year. But skipping out on travel may be a big mistake. Visiting new places not only provides us with some fun in the sun and pictures to share on social media, it also offers real health benefits that we may miss out on if we stay at home.

Of course taking a break from the daily grind can relieve some of the stress of everyday responsibilities, but traveling does more than provide a respite. In fact, studies show that those who travel have a more positive outlook on life than those who don't. Even better, traveling has been shown to decrease the risk of heart disease and brain disorders like dementia and Alzheimer's disease.

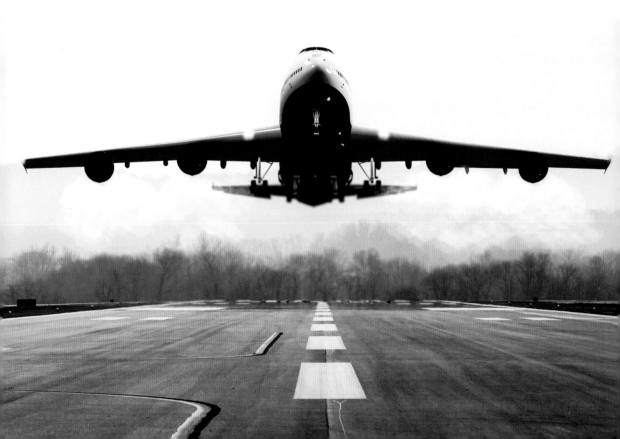

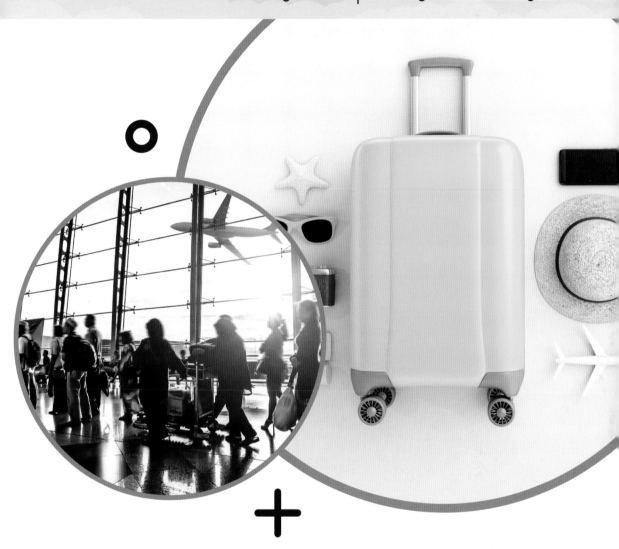

While there may be a few anxious moments during your wanderings—finding an affordable hotel, dealing with airport delays, waiting in lines—the positives outweigh the negatives. You don't even need to travel abroad (although it can be a definite plus!); taking a road trip or even visiting a new part of your own city can provide a brain boost. This is because new experiences directly affect the brain, causing it to work harder to process the foreign information. Learning about history and different cultures or trying new foods and experiences all give the brain a workout, prompting synapses to fire and boosting creativity and memory. Time to book that vacation!

5 Build a Birdhouse

Back in the 1800s, doctors would some-times prescribe an unusual treatment for women overcome with anxiety: knitting. While this "prescription" may seem like an antiquated idea, the unconventional treatment may have had basis in science. In fact, modern researchers have discov-ered that working with our hands can change the neurochemistry of the brain, increasing dopamine and serotonin and decreasing stress hormones.

What's more, using our hands—whether for something as simple as doodling or as complex as folding origami—has been shown to increase focus and im-prove memory. Experts even recommend taking notes by hand with good old pen and paper rather than typing them on a keyboard, as the action of writing long-hand improves memory retention.

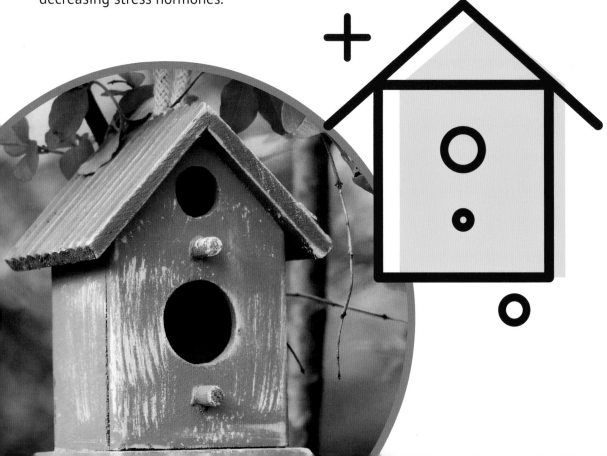

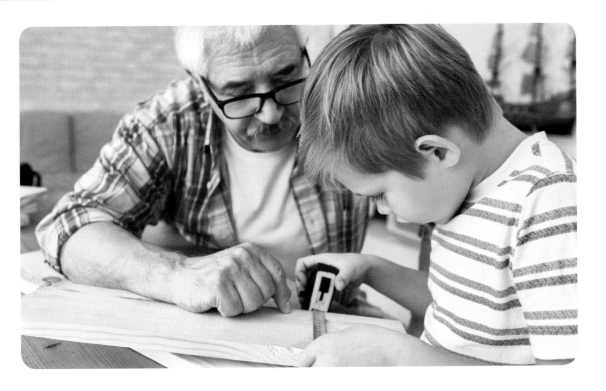

These kinds of activities often also result in a "reward," such as a knitted scarf, a handmade piece of pottery, or just a pile of neatly folded laundry, which adds to the beneficial neurochemicals in the brain. The act of physically working toward the reward gives us a sense of control that merely sitting at a desk or typing in an office environment doesn't provide. The brain is more engaged, attention is increased, and stress is lowered, which all add up to a better memory.

All kinds of hands-on activities can be beneficial, including needlepoint, woodworking, gardening, painting, cooking, metalworking, and sewing. The possibilities are endless, so try out a few new hobbies and see what you enjoy. You may even discover a hidden talent or two!

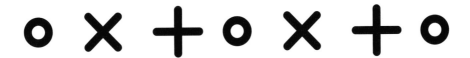

6 Clean Your Home

Even people who aren't ordinarily procrastinators can find it easy to put off household tasks while they pile up. Then one day we look around, and the work seems almost insurmountable, leading us to put it off for just one more day!

Between long hours at work, family commitments, hobbies, and time spent with friends, we're kept busy pretty much all day, every day. It's easy to neglect our home while dust, clutter, and dirt accumulate. Cleaning and maintaining our household, though, helps make it a soothing refuge when we need it most.

Your cleaning schedule for both regular and seasonal care should be organized in a way that makes you comfortable: You may choose to clean for an hour every morning, two hours after work, or all Saturday morning. As long as you have a schedule that leaves room for spontaneity, you'll stay ahead of housework.

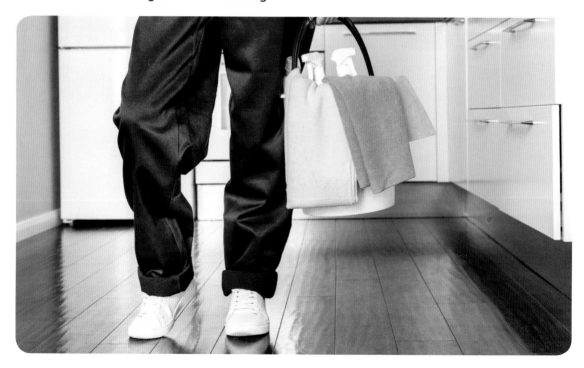

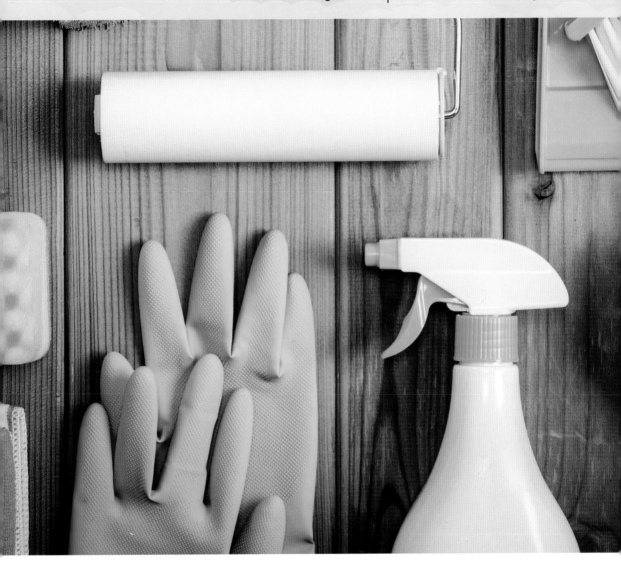

Basic day-to-day chores, such as beds, dishes, baths, laundry, and floor care, require a firm routine. Big tasks, such as closets, ovens, and silver, are often best tackled on impulse and require an elastic plan. If a big chore is hanging over your head and you keep putting it off, wait. It will be there when you are up to it, and you'll probably do a better job if you are ready to tackle it. Remember that when you are in the mood to clean, your cleaning tasks will get done much faster if there are no interruptions

7 Join a Gym

When we think of exercise, one of the images that pops into our head is that of muscle-bound, healthy people working out at the gym. If you don't have a gym membership, you may have wondered if you should get one. Not necessarily. If you dread the very thought, your chances of using the membership decrease.

For some people, a gym might be the right choice. Some people like the availability of different equipment they can try, or the idea of having a specific place to go at a specific time. If you do want to join a gym, here are some factors to consider:

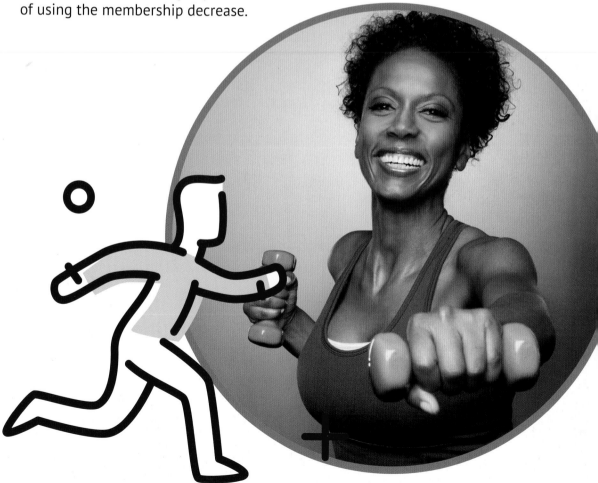

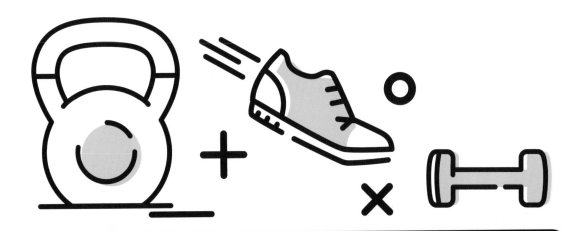

• What is the cost, and how are payments structured?

• How far away is the gym? Is it close to your workplace? Your home?

• When you talk to staff members, do they pressure you to join? If you ask for a tour, do they give you a thorough one?

• Can you get a free day pass? If so, go at the time you would usually want to go. How crowded is it? Do you have a long wait period for the machines you want to use? Are there any time limits on the popular machines? Are staff available to demonstrate how to use machines safely and effectively?

• Is the equipment clean? Are the showers and the locker room clean and well-maintained?

• Is the gym a chain? If so, can you go to any gym in the chain or only one location?

Before you commit to anything, ask friends about their gyms, and if you can, look online for reviews.

8 Strength Train

Strength training involves moderate to high exertion for short periods of time. When a muscle is worked to near (but not quite) exhaustion, the muscle becomes stronger and more efficient. Stronger and more efficient muscles burn more calories every minute of the day, whether you are actively working them or not, and they can help you achieve your weight loss goals more quickly. Other types of exercise will improve flexibility and balance. These are especially important as we age.

As with any form of exercise, when you start lifting weights, it is best to start very slow and easy; otherwise, you could wind up very sore and discouraged afterward. As time goes on, gradually increase the number of repetitions (reps) you do of each weight lifting exercise. Increase the amount of weight you use as well. Don't get discouraged if you reach a plateau and find it diffcult to increase the weight or do additional reps; everyone hits plateaus at some points. Just work on perfecting your technique.

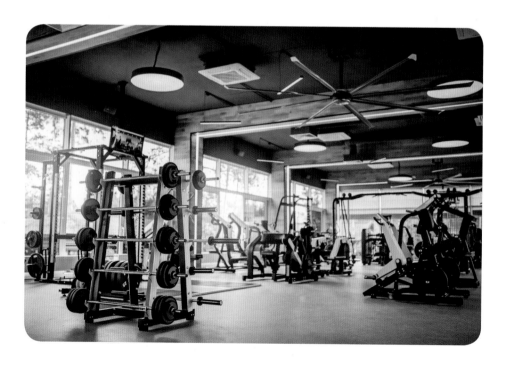

Here are some pointers to help make your weight-lifting workouts safer and more effective:

• Lift in the proper order. Start with exercises that work the big muscles in the chest, back, thighs, and shoulders, and end with lifts that train the smaller muscles of the arms and lower legs. When going through your lifting routine, try to alternate between exercises that work your arms and shoulders, those that strengthen your abdomen and lower back, and those that focus on your buttocks and legs.

• Never hold your breath when lifting weight. This can cause a dangerous rise in blood pressure. Blow air out when you raise the weight, and inhale as you lower it.

• Skip a day between weight-lifting workouts to give muscles time to recover and become stronger.

• Do not proceed until your technique is perfect. Be sure you can maintain the proper form for every single rep before you increase the weight or the number of reps. If you struggle with the last couple of reps, stay where you are until you can do them all properly.

• Lift and lower weight using slow, controlled movements. Slow lifts produce the best results.

9 Try Ball Exercises

The best part about ball exercises is that they are very low-impact and can be engaged in at whatever intensity level you are comfortable with. That means that you can scale up intensity at whatever pace works best for you.

Fitness ball workouts can also be incorporated into your daily routine, especially if you spend a lot of time sitting. Just swap out your office chair for a large fitness ball, and you can do exercises while you work. Ball workouts are particularly great for building your core strength.

The basic ball workout is to simply sit on the ball with your shoulders back and your core engaged, and simply bounce!

The key to this exercise is to bounce up rather than bounce down. Reach forward and back while you bounce, and vary bringing your arms in or out. You'll be amazed by what a difference this simple routine will have!

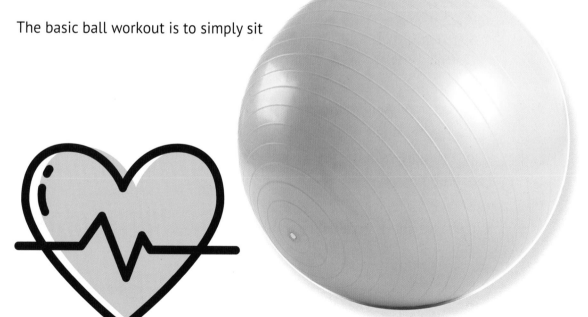

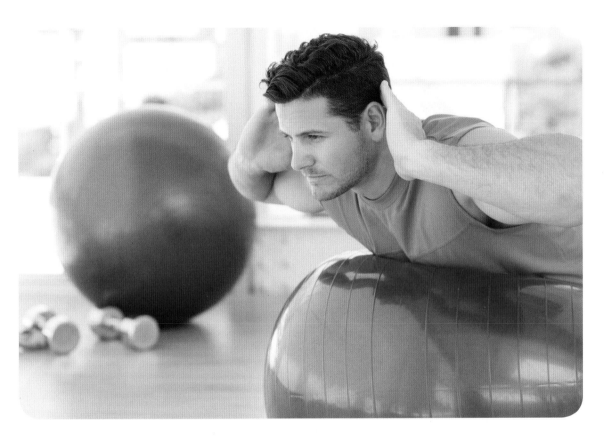

For more involved ball workouts, you can try different positions and routines. You can walk your legs out until your shoulders rest on the ball and your knees are at a ninety-degree angle. Extend your arms toward the ceiling, clasp your hands together, and engage your glutes. Walk your feet back as you move into a sitting position.

You can develop these exercises or make up your own that involve picking the ball up, bouncing on it in different ways, or using it as a support for other exercises. These exercises can also be made slightly more intensive by using three- or five-pound dumbbells to help tone your arm muscles while you engage your core. The important thing is to have fun with it!

10 Take a Walk

Walking is so simple that we often overlook it as a form of exercise. But it has a lot of advantages. You don't need fancy gear or equipment. It's low impact. And you can fit a brisk 10-minute (or longer) walk into your way of life more easily than almost any other kind of exercise.

Although not as strenuous as jogging, walking will increase your heart rate and oxygen consumption enough to qualify as an aerobic exercise. When you walk, your heart starts to beat faster and move larger amounts of oxygen-rich blood around your body more forcefully. Your blood vessels expand to carry this oxygen. In your working muscles, unused blood vessels open up to permit a good pickup of oxygen and release of carbon dioxide. These changes improve your ability to process oxygen. And better circulation to your leg muscles can mean less leg fatigue and fewer aches.

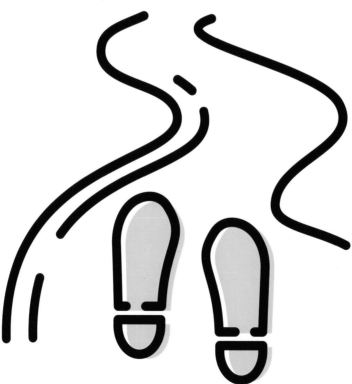

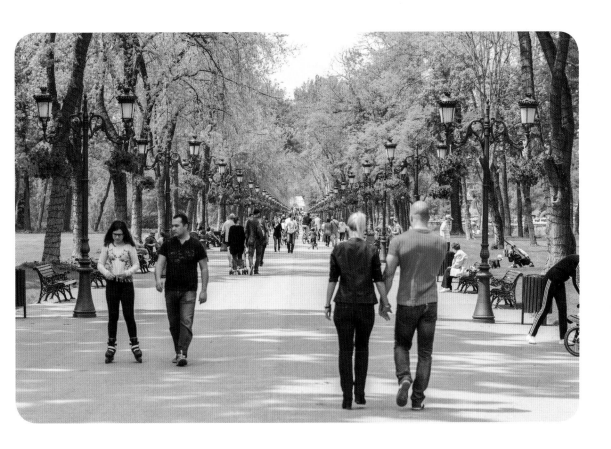

Walking indoors is also an option. If you walk on an indoor track, it is best to switch directions every other day. By walking counterclockwise one day and clockwise the next, you will help avoid orthopedic problems that can result from walking on a surface that slopes to the left or right. You can also try out a treadmill. (Don't buy a treadmill unless you've tried one out and know you'll use it, though! If you do decide to purchase one, it's a good idea to try it out in the store.)

The aerobic benefits aren't the only ones you'll get by incorporating walking into your life. Walking can refocus your attention from whatever is troubling you, reducing anxiety, tension, and stress. It helps you relax and recharge your mind and body.

11 Practice Yoga

Yoga, from India, is another of the world's oldest health practices that has the effects of elevating mood, reducing tension and fatigue, and putting people in a positive mood.

Although often associated with Eastern religions and practices, yoga is increasingly being adopted by Westerners for its numerous benefits. The most notable of these are increased circulation, better flexibility of muscles and joints, relaxation, and improved sleep.

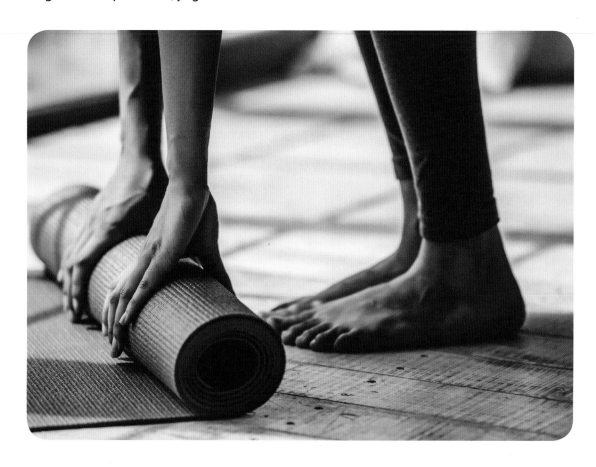

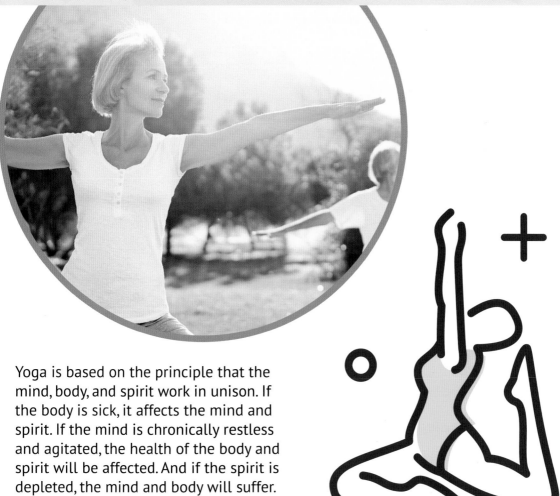

Yoga is based on the principle that the mind, body, and spirit work in unison. If the body is sick, it affects the mind and spirit. If the mind is chronically restless and agitated, the health of the body and spirit will be affected. And if the spirit is depleted, the mind and body will suffer. There are many forms of yoga, many of which use various poses that incorporate stretching and breathing exercises to integrate mind, body, and spirit. (Don't worry: You don't have to lay on a bed of nails or twist your body into a pretzel shape to achieve yoga's benefits.)

Yoga can help by loosening tight muscles, releasing tension, and putting you into a deep state of relaxation. But it's a type of relaxation that requires fixed attention to work well. The breathing and stretching exercises are designed to slow down your racing thoughts and pull you into the present moment. The practice of yoga helps stem the flow of stress hormones that your body produces when you are under stress. Indeed, when your body, mind, and spirit are connected and relaxed, you are more resilient to stress. You will also undoubtedly sleep better.

12 Try Tai Chi

Tai chi is an extremely interesting and enjoyable art to practice. And requirements for equipment and space are absolutely minimal: Tai chi can be practiced almost anywhere that a few square yards of space are available. Most importantly, its health benefits are readily apparent to practitioners from the very beginning of training.

Tai chi is a gentle art, so gentle that people of almost any age or physical condition can undertake it. In fact, many prominent teachers began their careers teaching tai chi late in life.

Today, many different types of tai chi organizations have sprung up, each specializing in unique forms. Some of these groups have even designed instructional techniques specifically for older people, and private research centers now study the healing effects of tai chi.

Tai chi's fluid movements, always spiraling and bending, actually massage the internal organs, releasing them from damaging constrictions brought about by such factors as stress, poor posture, and difficult working conditions. This is one of the main health benefits of practicing tai chi. Some of the other purported benefits of regular tai chi practice that are currently under investigation include improved circulation, breathing, digestion, and flexion of limbs; stress management; relief from high blood pressure, back pain, and insomnia; and better overall health.

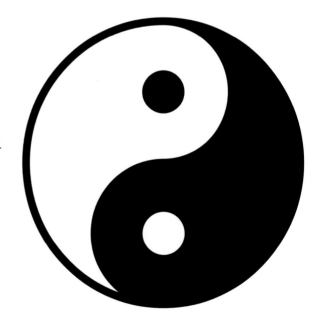

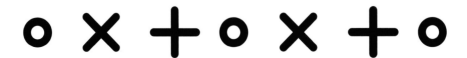

In fact, one study which examined the effects of tai chi on the elderly found that only 15 minutes of daily tai chi practice could significantly reduce the number of fall-related injuries.

At present, billions of medical dollars are spent annually caring for the elderly after injuries of this type. Couple this figure with the pain and inconvenience suffered by the victims, and one has a very good reason to promote tai chi!

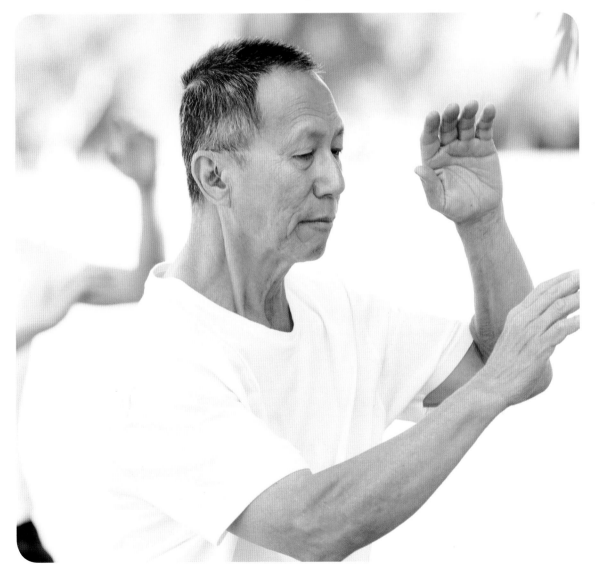

13 Go Dancing

Dancing is another really fun way to get exercise, release tension, and relieve stress.

Whether you decide to dance alone in your own living room, take dance lessons with a friend or significant other, or even go to a club dance hall, you can enjoy all of the wonderful benefits of dancing whenever you like.

A huge additional benefit to dancing is that as you get better at it, you'll find yourself getting more comfortable with your own body. That leads to more self-confidence and esteem, which will only encourage you to dance more!

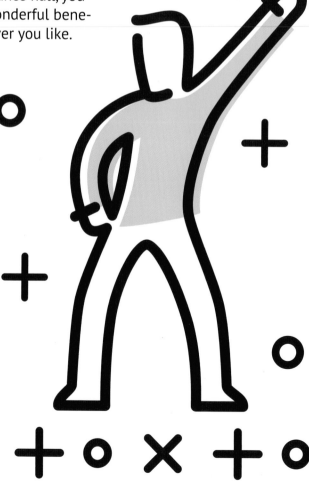

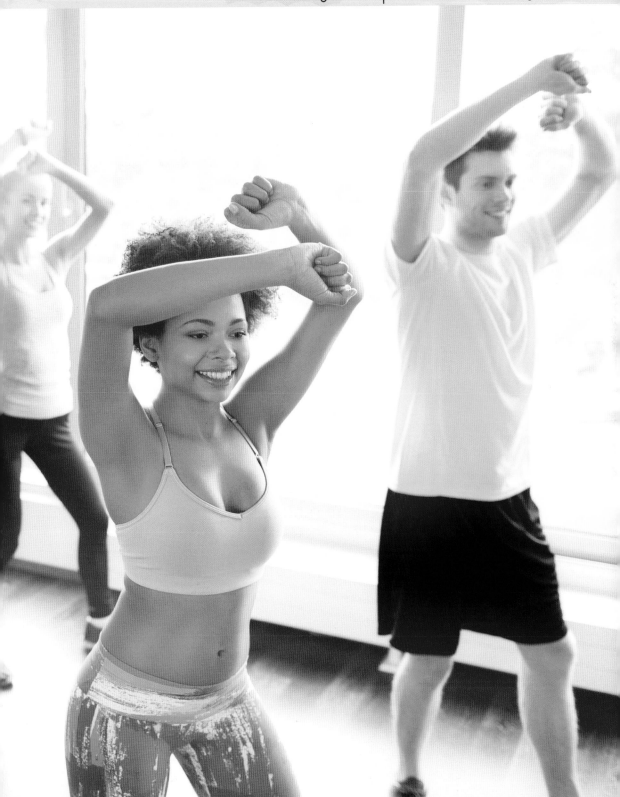

14 Bicycle

Whether you're on a stationary bicycle or outdoors, bicycling is one of the best cardio workouts that also burns calories and is low-impact.

One of the reasons bicycling is such an excellent cardio workout is because you can incorporate it into your daily routine. You can ride your bicycle to the market or to run errands around the neighborhood. You can ride a commuter bike to and from work. You can ride with friends and family on weekends to go to the beach, to the park, to museums (where you'll get a great low intensity cardio workout walking around!), or anywhere else you typically take your car or ride the bus. And because cycling is so low-impact, it is easy on your joints and is an excellent cross-training exercise for aerobics or other high-impact exercises.

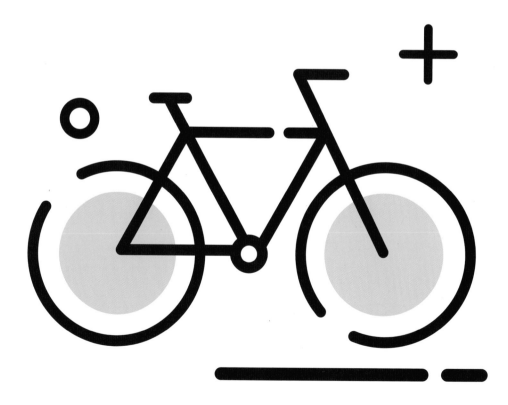

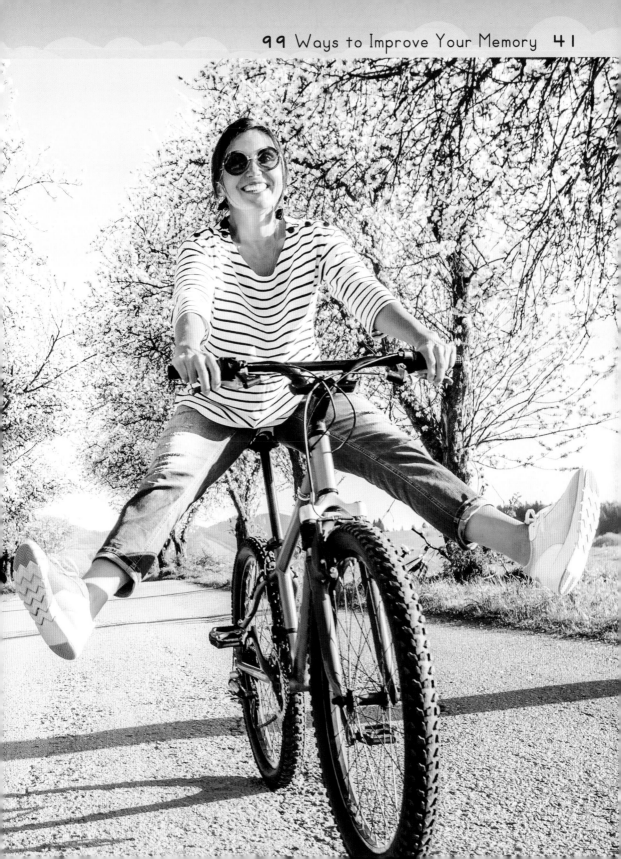

15 Swim!

This low-impact activity is not only superb for those with heightened exposure to injury, but it's also an excellent way to reduce stress levels and boost mood and brainpower. It increases blood flow, which in turn can improve cognition.

Swimming's physical benefits are plentiful. It's easy on the joints, improves flexibility, and strengthens the back and abdominal muscles. This is good news for those with chronic illnesses like arthritis or multiple sclerosis, since the activity eliminates the pain involved with weight-bearing exercises. In addition, swimming is a fantastic activity for cardiovascular health, as it improves circulation and lowers blood pressure. Swimmers also have better coordination and motor skills.

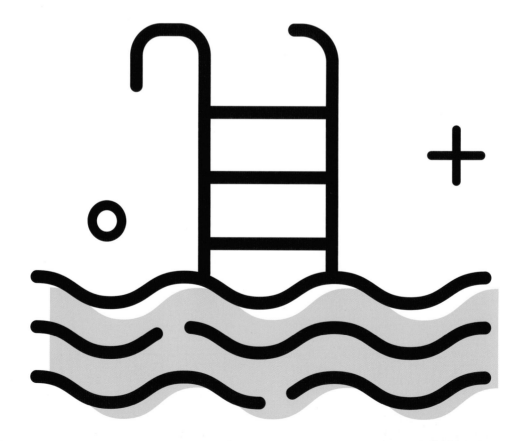

The psychological benefits of swimming are as numerous as the physical ones. It can lower depression (thanks, in part, to the release of dopamine, serotonin, and norepinephrine) and curtail anxiety. It can also be a social activity: swimming classes, or other aerobic activities and games, are staples of community pools, sports clubs, and gyms. Socializing, as we know, is essential for a healthy brain.

And most of all? Swimming is fun! Whether it's simple laps at the pool or aerobic exercises and games, swimming is an excellent activity for both physical and mental health. Get your bathing suit and take a dip!

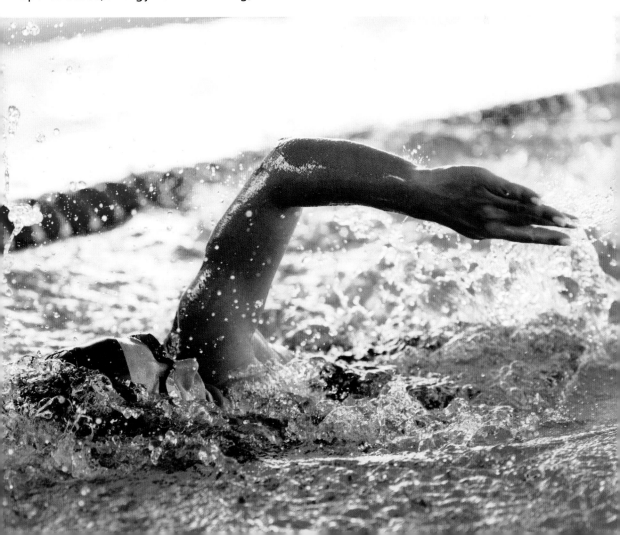

16 Garden

Gardening and outdoors work make for great physical activity that is rewarding for both the body and mind.

There's no doubt about it—gardening takes work. But the payback is immeasurable when you develop your property into a comfortable outdoor living area. The yard or garden is an extension of your home and yourself—with your signature in every detail. And building a harmonious space for leisure and function can be easier than you think. You can rely on trees and shrubs with interesting year-round characteristics and long-living perennials and bulbs to set the framework for an ever-changing landscape. You'll be able to have lush borders with continual bloom that are practically self-maintaining.

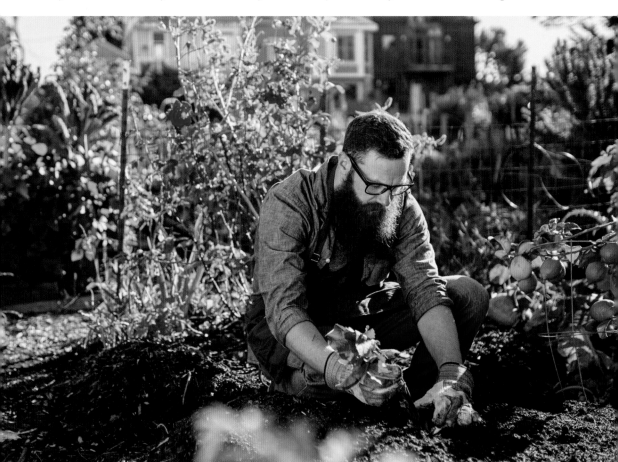

o x + o x + o

Some of the work may seem to be labor intensive, but the return on your initial investment will be appreciated for years to come. Your garden should require minimal tending while keeping an artistic flair. Gardening can be fun and even simple, without the drudgery of daily watering, weeding, and grooming. Indeed, by focusing just a little extra attention on fundamental things like soil, water, and light, you can make a major difference in your garden.

But perhaps best of all, regular gardening promotes a variety of health benefits, according to AARP. It can lower dementia risks, fight stress, and combat loneliness. That's not to mention the aerobic exercise benefits and the added bonus of Vitamin D thanks to sunlight exposure.

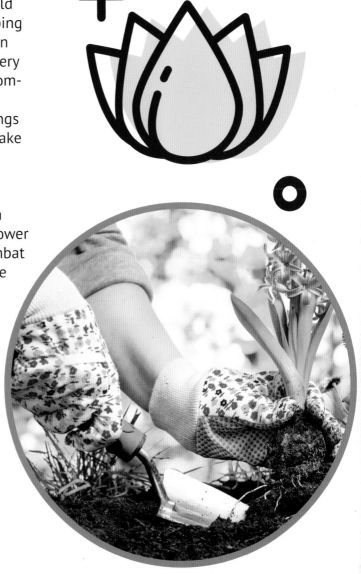

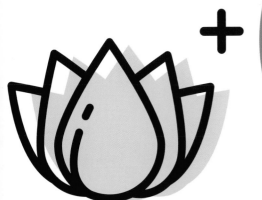

17 Use Mnemonic Devices

If you ever learned the name "Roy G. Biv" to remember the colors of the rainbow (red, orange, yellow, green, blue, indigo, and violet), you're familiar with the idea of a mnemonic device. Mnemonics often use phrases, acronyms, rhymes, or visual imagery to help with the recollection of larger pieces of information. Their effectiveness has been well-documented, with studies showing that mnemonic devices are especially helpful to those with memory deficits caused by neurological conditions and those with weak long-term memory.

Mnemonic devices aren't new; in fact, ancient Greeks and Romans were fond of using the "method of loci" or the "mind palace technique" to help with recollection of information. In this method, a familiar location, such as a home or a daily route to work, is imagined, with the information that needs to be remembered assigned to different rooms or landmarks. The information is then mentally associated with specific locations, making it easier to recall at a later time.

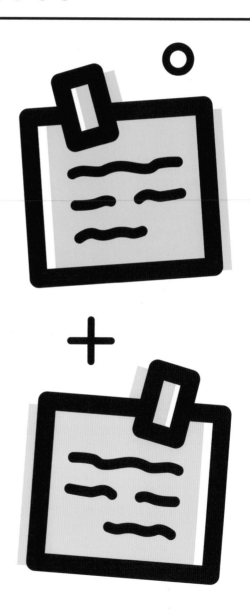

Other mnemonics include name mnemonics, such as the colorful "Roy G. Biv," music, like the ABC song we all remember from childhood, and rhymes, like the familiar "In 1492, Columbus sailed the ocean blue." All of these methods work by making the information more meaningful or by giving it a more organized structure.

These are just a few of the mnemonic devices that can make remembering lists and tasks easier. To explore more of the fun and clever ways these methods can be used, visit www.verywellhealth.com and search for "mnemonics."

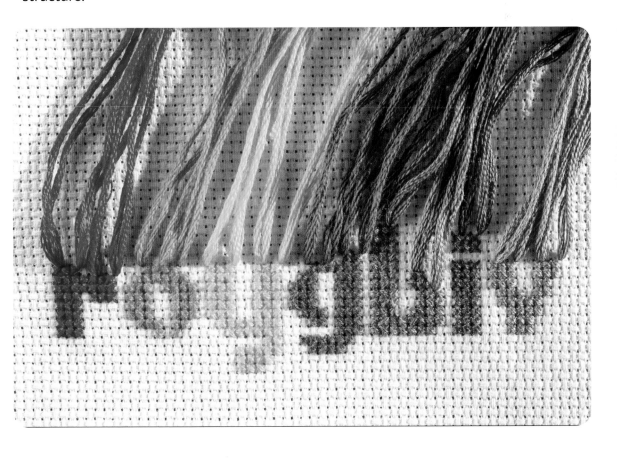

18 Learn a Language

If you've ever considered learning a new language but thought you were "too old" to tackle such an endeavor, think again. Researchers have discovered that learning a new language at any age can have major brain benefits.

The effects of learning a language on children have been widely studied, with researchers proving that bilingual children perform better at tasks using memory skills than their monolingual counterparts. But recently, scientists have been studying the effects of learning a new language on older brains, and it turns out that the same holds true for adults, as well.

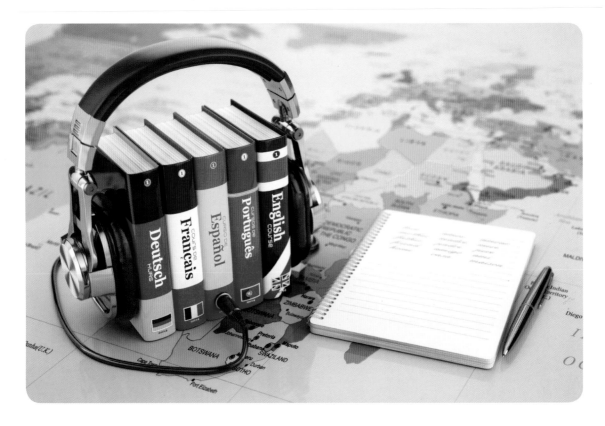

One study showed that the effort of learning a new language trains the brain to switch back and forth between languages, which improves a mechanism in the brain that controls concentration. In fact, drugs designed to slow the progression of Alzheimer's disease target this same mechanism, and those who speak more than one language are less likely to be afflicted with the brain disorder. Brain scans of those who learn languages show an increase in the size of the hippocampus, the area of the brain responsible for storing and retrieving memories.

Besides improving memory and staving off Alzheimer's disease, learning a new language comes with a myriad of benefits, including better focus, smarter decision-making, and improved creativity.

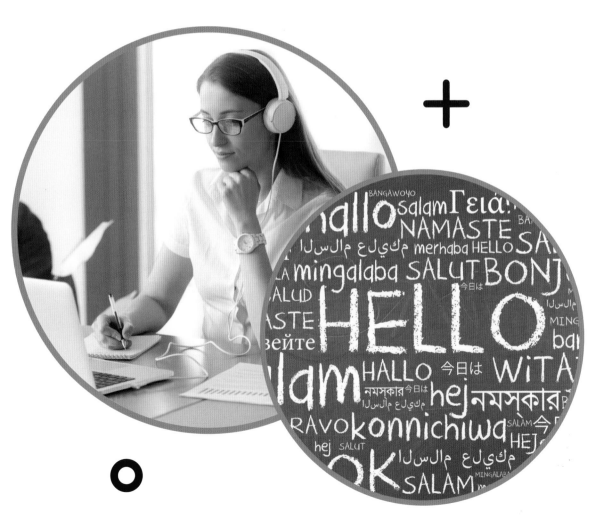

19 Visit a Museum or Art Gallery

The love of art is subjective. Some appreciate the brushstrokes of Renaissance masters like Michelangelo and Botticelli, while others are drawn toward the modern flair of Picasso or Matisse. But no matter what kind of art you enjoy, one thing is certain: visiting a museum is greatly beneficial for your brain.

Scientists have discovered that those who visit museums or art galleries, even for as little as 30 minutes, show a decrease in the stress hormone cortisol, and an increase in beneficial brain chemicals. In one study, in which volunteers viewed art while neurobiologists scanned their brains, researchers discovered that looking at art caused an increase in dopamine, the same chemical related to feelings of love. It also resulted in a 10 percent increase in blood flow to the brain, a phenomenon related to—guess what?—falling in love. It would seem that art and love are closely related!

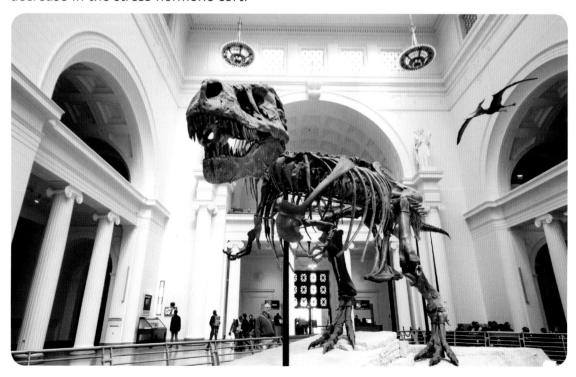

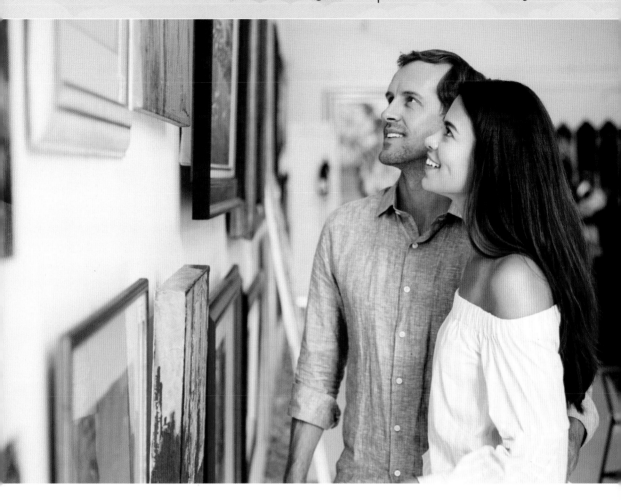

But viewing art does more than provide us with fuzzy, warm feelings. Wandering through a museum engages the brain in a complex activity, as it takes in new sights and processes the information. While it does so, it creates new neural connections, causing better communication between the right and left hemisphere of the brain. All of this results in reduced stress, stronger critical thinking skills, and a better memory. In fact, people with dementia or Alzheimer's disease who frequently participate in visual arts activities often see great improvement of their symptoms. While art itself may be subjective, the benefits that come from viewing it are certainly not.

o x + o x + o

20 Plot Your Family Tree

There are many things we all strive to remember on a regular basis, such as shopping lists, where we left our sunglasses, and whether we took daily medication. But thinking of family stories and history is much more meaningful than the daily tasks on our minds. That's one reason that plotting a family tree can provide a boost for your brain.

In fact, experts say that thinking about fond old memories can have a "cinematic" quality, activating areas of the brain that not only recall the moment in time, but also the smells, sounds, and sights that went along with it. These memories can play out in the mind like an old film, with pieces of the recollection forming together like a puzzle in the brain.

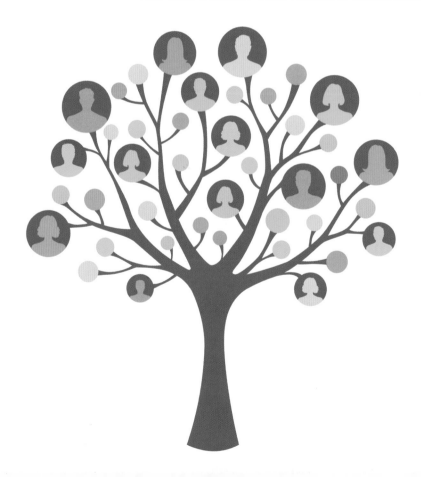

When we first experience a major life event, such as a wedding or the birth of a child, the specific unique aspects of that event are stored in different areas of the brain. Later, when we recall the moment, the hippocampus is able to trigger each of these areas in the brain to activate, giving us a clear picture of the past.

Constructing a family tree does more than activate old memories. The process also requires research and organization, as you search through pictures, records, and letters to build the branches of your ancestry. It's a workout for your brain!

Try too making a "concentration"-like memory game using pictures of ancestors and playing with some of members of the younger generation. Every match will provide a new story to tell, ensuring family history is passed down.

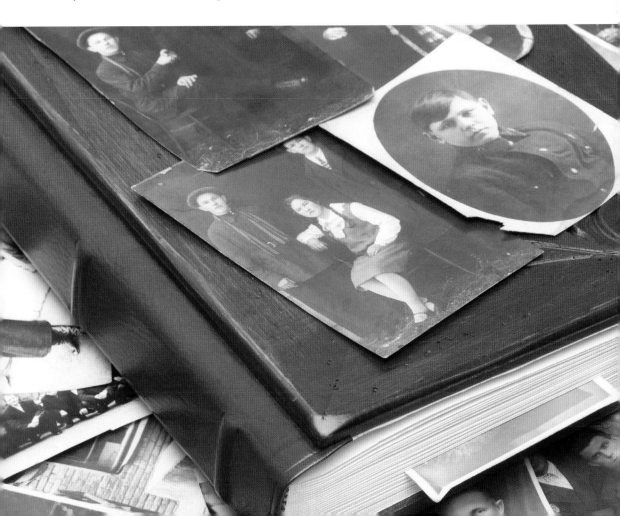

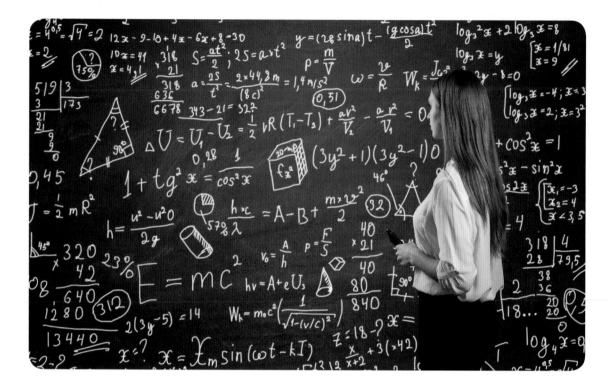

21 (Re)-learn Mathematics

Some of us may shudder at the idea of delving into mathematics after decades of being away from school. Multiplication, division, fractions, formulas—if we're not using them "in real life," what good are they? As it turns out, learning math skills does more than help us count correct change; it can provide major brain benefits, as well.

Math is especially helpful for improving short-term memory, or "working memory," which is the information we hold in our minds at any given moment. Only a small amount of information can be held in our working memory, and usually only for a few seconds at a time. So if it becomes overwhelmed, even simple thought processes can seem complex, as our brains work backwards and forwards searching for answers.

But scientists have discovered that practicing mathematics engages our working memory. And the more it is used, the more efficient working memory becomes. The mental exercise of practicing and mastering math problems helps to free up this memory, which in turn also improves focus and concentration. Learning mathematics has also been shown to improve "implicit memory," which is the unconscious memory of deeply imbedded skills, such as riding a bike, driving a car, or playing an instrument.

To give your brain a mathematical workout, seek out websites where you can take some free lessons.

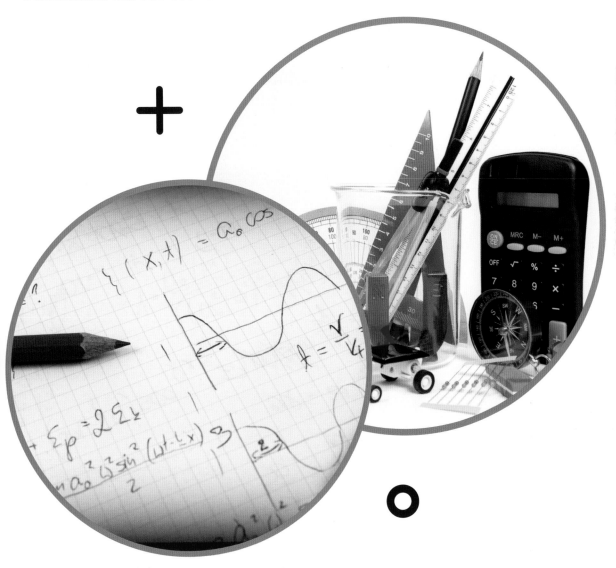

22 Make a Scrapbook

These days, many of us keep all of our photos on our smartphones, where we can scroll through them to quickly reminisce or post them to social media to share with family and friends. But smartphones are a fairly recent invention; before they became commonplace, people still wanted a way to keep all their memories—including recipes, letters, and other memorabilia—in one place. What better way to accomplish this than with a scrapbook?

Scrapbooking officially began in the United Kingdom in the nineteenth century, but even before this hobby had a name, people were collecting memorabilia and placing it in books and albums. The concept grew over the centuries, and by the early 2000s, scrapbooking was a multibillion-dollar industry. Nowadays, scrapbooking has evolved to include digital scrapbooking, where entire albums are created online.

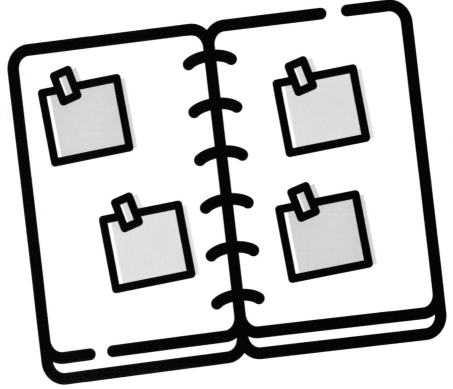

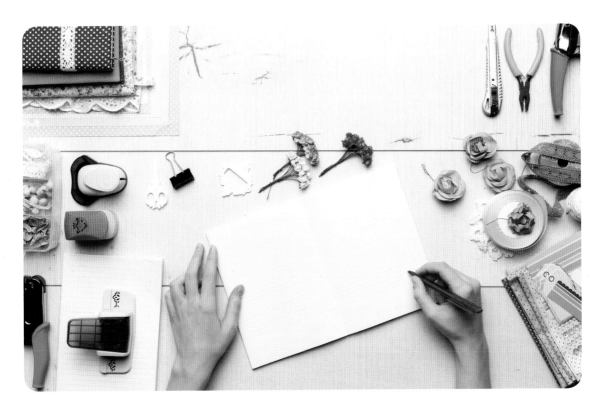

But this time-honored tradition is more than just big business. Scrapbooking provides some major cognitive benefits, as well. The simple process of sorting through pictures, cards, and documents stimulates the brain to recall long-forgotten memories. What's more, assembling a scrapbook is an artistic endeavor, and learning creative skills has been shown to boost short-term memory.

Scrapbooking has also been shown to reduce stress, which can contribute to memory problems. There has even been evidence that scrapbooking with those afflicted with dementia or Alzheimer's can help stir up past memories, even in those with advanced cases of disease.

Storing all of our memories on a phone may be convenient, but perhaps it's time to get those creative juices flowing and see what sorts of memories you can unlock with the meaningful and rewarding art of scrapbooking.

23 Keep a Calendar

When it comes to tips for a better memory, one word pops up on experts' lists of suggestions more than any other: organization. And it makes sense; after all, when your home or office are in disarray, your mind tends to follow suit. Short-term memory, also called working memory, retrieves information from readily available sources, from either what is already in your memory, or from real-world experience like a conversation or reading material. So if you're constantly forced to search for dates or times on sticky notes or in note pads, the efficiency of your working memory is interrupted.

Working memory also has a very limited capacity, with most experts believing that our minds can only hold, at most, around seven items of new information at time. And, unless we actively attend to it or rehearse it, that information only stays in our memory for 10 to 15 seconds. It takes a lot of effort to keep items in our memory for a longer time, which can leave us feeling cognitively overwhelmed.

To ensure that working memory moves along coherently and to prevent feeling overwhelmed, organization is key. And there's no easier way to stay organized than by keeping a calendar.

Writing down events, appointments, and important dates on a calendar or in an electronic planner consolidates information in one easily accessible location. Make it a habit to consult your calendar several times a day, and you'll always feel like you're on top of your schedule.

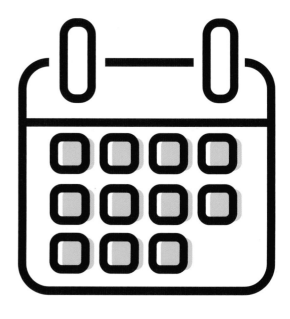

24 Practice Positive Thinking

Some of us have that one person in our lives who seems to be in a perpetual good mood. No matter the circumstances, they're always able to look on the bright side, seeing the glass as half full even when the rest of us are brooding in the dark. Or maybe you are that person—optimistic and chipper, giving family, friends, and co-workers pep talks when troubles arise. If that sounds like you, give yourself a pat on the back—because in addition to making others happy, you're making your brain happy, as well.

Positive and negative thoughts each affect the brain in different ways. Anxious, stressful, or angry thoughts overwork the prefrontal cortex of the brain, which results in a brain that is unable to work at its normal capacity. The ability to think literally slows down, making it difficult to process information.

Happy or optimistic thoughts, on the other hand, actually enhance the function of the prefrontal cortex, causing brain growth in this area. The result is greater cognitive flexibility, enhanced creativity, a better ability to analyze, and faster thought processing. And interestingly, having a positive outlook can affect how we later recall a situation. Thinking optimistically before a life event—even if that event is negative—causes the memory of the event to be remembered more favorably.

It's not easy to simply be optimistic if your natural tendency is pessimism. But experts recommend avoiding negative self-talk, seeking out sources of humor, and making the effort to practice positive thinking on a daily basis.

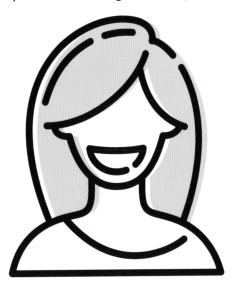

25 Make To-Do Lists (and Other Lists)

Life can be overwhelming at times. Between work meetings, school functions, doctor's appointments, family get-togethers, and a myriad of other events, our days are often jam-packed. Add in things like grocery shopping, cleaning out the garage, tending to the garden, and doing laundry, and it can be difficult to remember what needs to be done and when.

Fortunately, a simple to-do list may be all the help you need. The act of writing, especially by hand, forces your brain to work a bit harder, helping you to remember items on your list even when you're not reading it. This is true for other lists as well, such as shopping lists or lists of items you need to pack for a vacation. Writing down each item can make it much easier to recall later on, even if your list isn't in front of you.

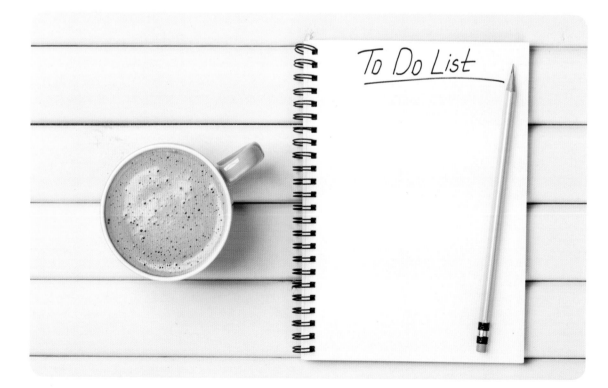

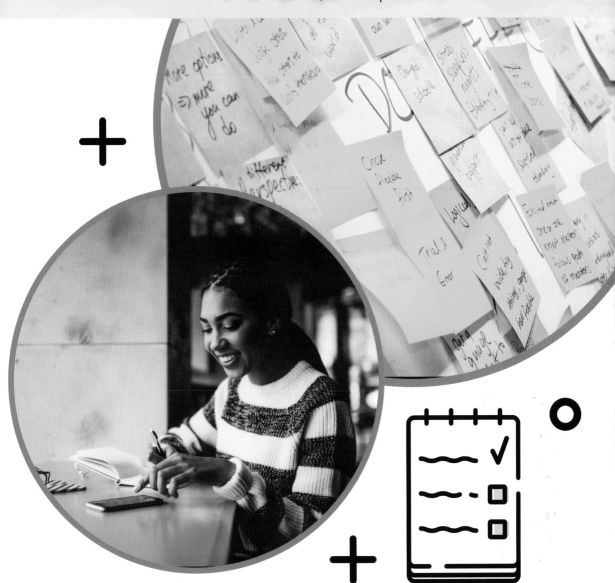

Writing out a to-do list also makes abstract ideas seem more concrete. Perhaps you've been thinking about organizing the pantry for weeks, but the thought keeps slipping your mind. Writing it down on a to-do list gives you a concrete goal, making it much more probable that you'll tackle the task.

Making a to-do list is a simple way to outline tasks, prevent anxiety, and provide proof of what we've accomplished. In fact, even if you don't finish everything on the list, writing a to-do list gives your brain a mental boost.

26 Learn an Instrument

If you were like many children, you may have taken musical instrument lessons when you were young. Piano, guitar, violin—many of us have memories of practicing our chosen instrument (but not always successfully). Learning an instrument as a child is quite a common occurrence in the U.S.; in fact, in a survey of households with members who play instruments, more than 60 percent of those surveyed began lessons between the ages of 5 and 11.

Studies show that children who take music lessons have better spatial-temporal skills than their non-musical counterparts. But it would be a mistake to think that the benefits of learning an instrument only apply to children. In fact, the benefits of playing a musical instrument have been proven to span all age groups.

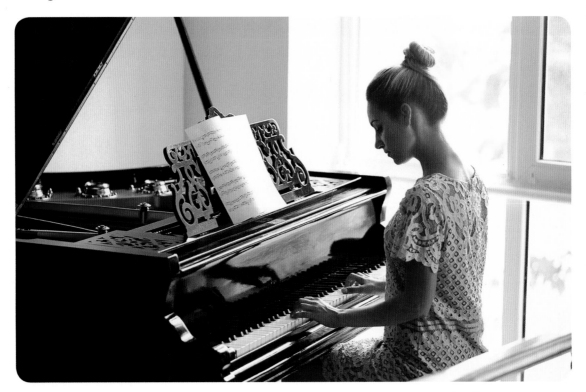

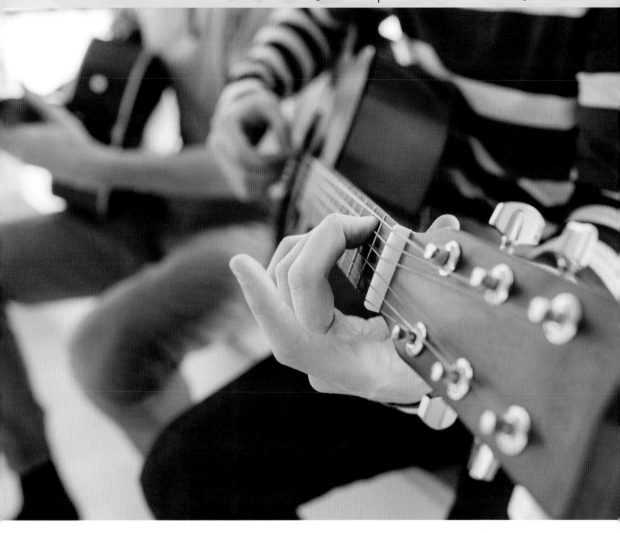

Learning a musical instrument provides some unique benefits, since music influences parts of the brain that other stimuli don't. It helps to increase gray matter volume in these areas, and it strengthens the connections between them. Although the areas of the brain that process music see the greatest benefit, learning an instrument also enhances verbal memory, spatial reasoning, emotion, and auditory processing. And since it requires a high working memory load, playing an instrument increases memory capacity.

There's even evidence that learning a musical instrument can increase your IQ score by an average of seven points!

27 Explore Brain Stimulation

The idea of zapping the brain with electrical currents sounds like something out of a science fiction movie. But surprisingly, noninvasive brain stimulation is already a reality that is showing some real promise for turning back the clock on aging brains.

A recent study lead by Boston University neuroscientists Robert Reinhart and John Nguyen used electroencephalography (EEG)—a way to monitor electrical activity in the brain using electrodes placed along the scalp—to monitor and stimulate the brains of study participants. Their research focused on working memory in two groups of adults: one group was between the ages of 20 and 29, and the other was between the ages of 60 and 76.

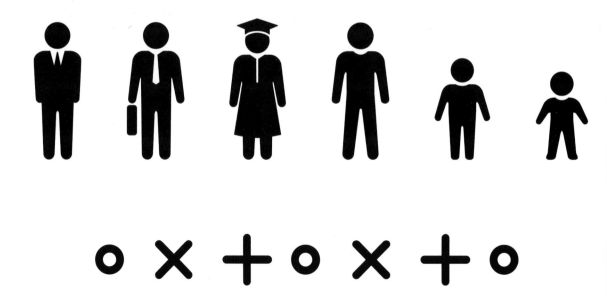

Reinhart and Nguyen had the volunteers perform a working memory task while monitoring their brain activity. As the efficiency of working memory declines throughout adulthood, the older participants performed, on average, about 10 percent less accurately than their younger counterparts. But when the scientists pulsed electrical stimulation through the prefrontal and temporal areas of the volunteers' brains, the older adults began to perform just as well as the younger group. What's more, when Reinhart and Nguyen tried the same brain stimulation on the poorest-performing members of the young group, their scores improved as well.

Although brain stimulation is still in its experimental stage, the findings of the study were so promising that scientists are confident that the technique can soon be used for patients suffering from memory disorders.

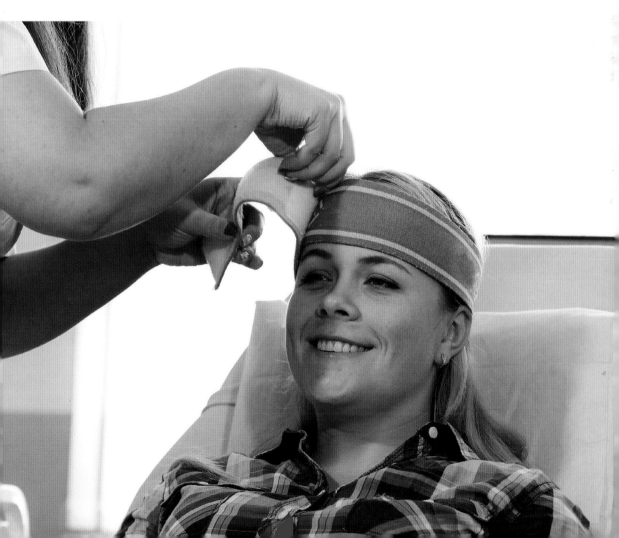

28 Listen to Classical Music

The idea of "the Mozart Effect" has been around at least since the early 1990s, when a psychologist demonstrated that college kids who listened to the composer's music before a test performed better. Although it was one small study, the idea that listening to Mozart could make kids smarter took on a life of its own. Soon, parents were encouraging younger and younger children to listen to classical music. Today, albums with titles like "Brilliant Babies," "Beethoven for Babies," and even "Mozart for Mothers-to-be" are marketed to parents of newborns, who hope their little ones will start their lives with a musical brain boost.

And it turns out that there may be some truth to "the Mozart Effect," even for those of us who have reached adulthood. In fact, recent research has gone all the way to the molecular level to unlock the secrets of this effect. Scientists studied blood samples from volunteers who either listened to classical music or no music, and then studied the genes of each group. Those who listened to the music showed enhanced activity in genes responsible for synaptic function, learning, and memory.

In another study, students listened to a lecture, either with classical music playing in the background or with no music. When the two groups were later quizzed on the lecture, those who had heard the classical music scored better than the no-music group.

Clearly, classical music has a positive effect on the brain, whether you're a child or an adult. Don't let the kids have all the fun—start reaping the benefits of "the Mozart Effect" yourself!

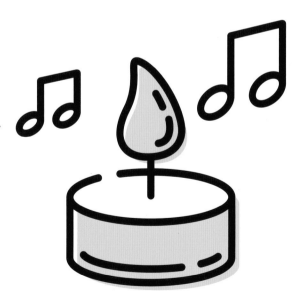

29 Play a Board Game

If you're like most of us, you probably have a few board games collecting dust in a closet somewhere. Chess, checkers, Monopoly, Scrabble—we've all played a game or two in our lives, but they often only see the light of day during family get-togethers or when the electricity goes out and television is no longer an option.

But board games, played at any age, provide some surprising brain benefits. In fact, the very nature of many of these games is conducive to better brain function. After all, many games require a good memory, problem-solving skills, and an ability to process complex situations. The more you play these games, the more you build up the hippocampus and prefrontal cortex, the areas of the brain responsible for complex functions. Like exercise for the brain, board games result in a sharper memory, improved learning capacity, and better cognitive function.

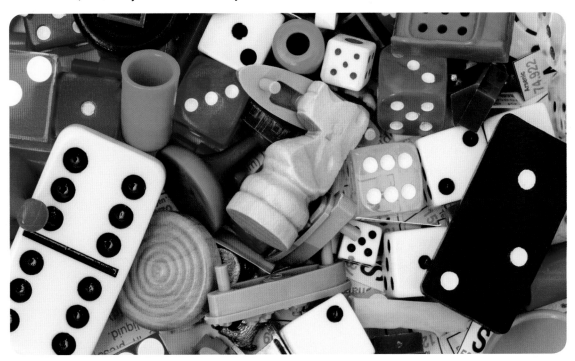

30 Learn How to Weave

People who suffer from stress, depression, or anxiety often look for ways to deal with their negative emotions. While therapy and medication can certainly help, some have found a surprisingly creative way to cope with unwanted feelings: crafting. Crafts like knitting, weaving, crocheting, and needlework have been proven to ease stress and even relieve chronic pain. The repetitive action and ever-changing skill level of these activities help crafters enter what psychologists call a "flow" state, or an immersive mindset balanced between skill and challenge. Providing a way to destress and relieve depression or anxiety is a huge benefit in its own right; but did you know that crafting can also protect your brain from damage caused by aging?

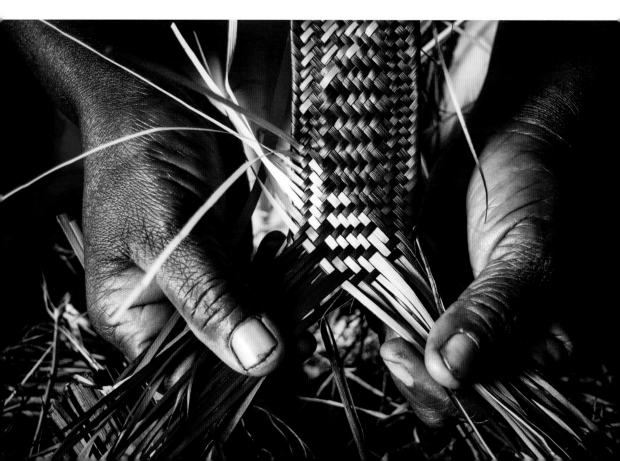

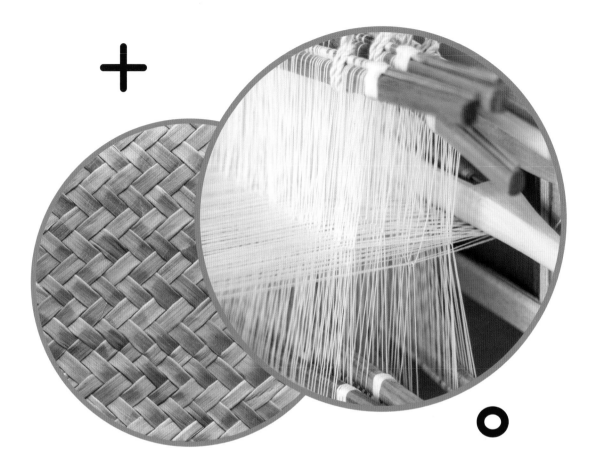

An international survey of thousands of crafters found that those who participate in a textile-based activity (like knitting or weaving) on a regular basis report improved cognitive abilities, including better memory, concentration, and problem-solving skills. The "flow" state may have something to do with it, as our brains are only capable of processing a certain amount of information at any given time. By entering this almost meditative state, the brain has the opportunity to rest and recoup.

What's more, learning a new skill improves the brain's processing speed and prevents cerebral atrophy, helping to fend off dementia. In fact, those who participate in crafting activities can reduce their chances of experiencing cognitive impairment by up to 50 percent. So why not weave some crafting into your life?

31 Play a Brain Training Computer Game

Computers have become a major part of our lives. We use them to work, stay connected to family and friends, research the best vacation spots, take notes, order groceries, and perform dozens of other helpful tasks. In fact, your home computer may even be able to help you improve your memory—and have fun at the same time.

"Brain training" has become a big trend in the U.S., with companies like Cogmed, WordSmart Corporation, and LearningRx growing into multibillion-dollar endeavors over the last two decades. The idea behind brain training is that by playing specially designed computer games on a regular basis, players can enhance their memories and improve their thinking skills. These games include puzzles and exercises that help to improve working memory, increase attention span, and enhance focus and brain speed.

Although there has been controversy over whether brain training can make you "smarter," scientists agree that these sorts of games can help prevent dementia and Alzheimer's disease. In studies of adults with mild cognitive impairment, brain training was shown to improve memory, attention, mood, and even self-perceived quality of life, leading researchers to conclude that playing these games reduces early symptoms of memory loss and can help maintain or even improve cognitive skills among older adults who are at risk of dementia.

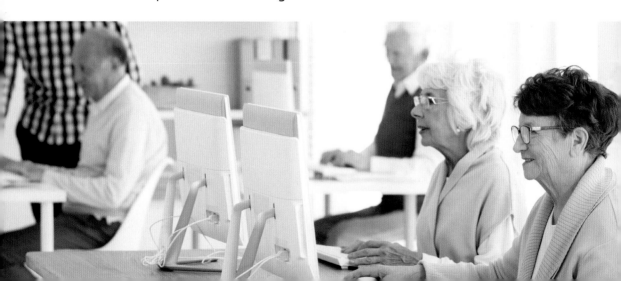

32 Learn Computer Programming

For many of today's adults, coding was and is a mysterious process. People might have learned the basics of BASIC in a computer lab, but they left the hard stuff to programmers. But with the explosion of smartphones and tablets, the ubiquity of the Internet, and an array of new programming languages, today's kids often have more opportunities to learn to code and to use these skills to create impressive animated stories and games. The skills they learn in terms of problem solving and logical thinking can help them in other areas of their life, too.

There are almost countless programming languages. Python, Java, and Ruby are some others that are used in a lot of offices. When we say these are "languages," it means something different than how Spanish, English, and Mandarin are languages. There is a list of terms—words, abbreviations, and other things, so not only dictionary words—and your computer knows that each term means the computer should do something.

Like brain training games, learning the fundamentals of computer programming can help improve thinking skills, which in turn boosts focus, memory, and brain speed. There are a wealth of online resources available to help understand programming languages. While initially intimidating, getting a grip on the basics of programming can be a liberating adventure!

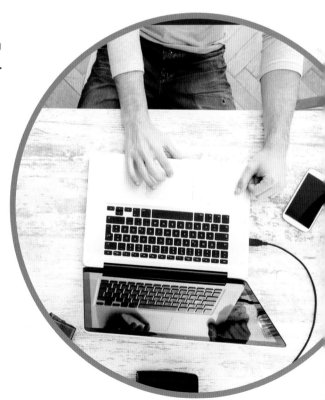

33 Turn Off Your GPS

Navigation programs, or global positioning systems (GPS), can be enormously helpful at times. Using GPS to find an unfamiliar address can alleviate some of the stress of driving, by planning out a route for you and prompting you to turn before you accidentally drive in the wrong direction. But surprisingly, this technology may not be as helpful as we think; in fact, it could be harming our brains.

A study looked into the effects on the brain of using GPS, and found that when we follow the instructions given by a navigation system, our brains don't need to work as hard as they would if we planned the route ourselves. Over time, this lack of usage in the "navigation" area of the brain—which is located in the hippocampus—could literally make finding our way in the world more difficult.

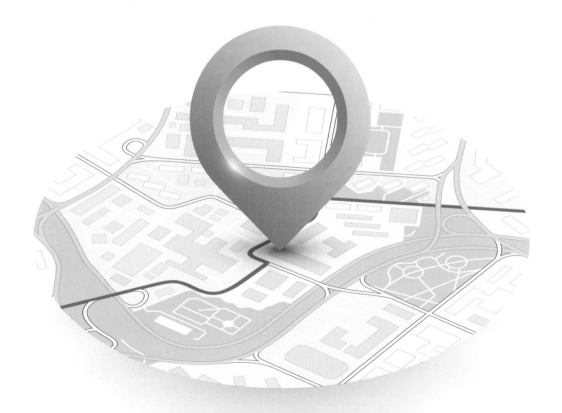

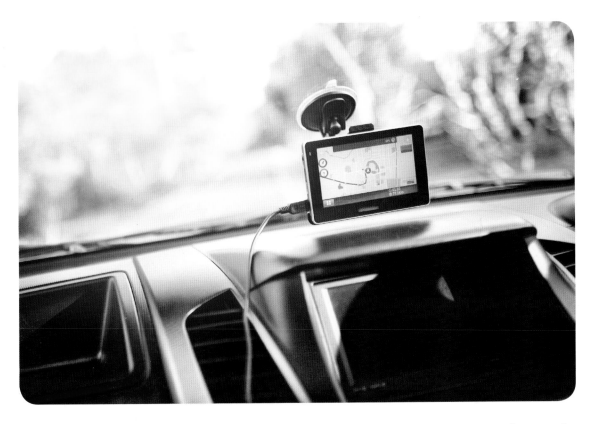

The study asked participants to find their way to a destination either by planning the route themselves or by using a GPS, while researchers tracked their brain activity. The results proved that those who navigated on their own had increased brain activity in the hippocampus, while those who used GPS had little activity in this region. Since the hippocampus is also involved in memory function, the more we use it the better our chance of retaining memories.

Scientists are concerned that our reliance on navigation systems is changing our brains, and not necessarily for the better. So the next time you're traveling, try switching off the GPS and taking an old-school approach to navigation.

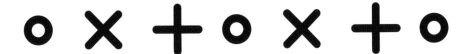

34 Paint a Picture

When we look at art, our brains are flooded with feel-good chemicals like dopamine, and neural connections within the brain are strengthened. But creating art benefits our brains even if we think we have zero artistic talent!

A study divided volunteers into two groups: one group took an art apprecia-tion class while the other simply painted and drew their own art. After 10 weeks, the group that created art showed positive changes in areas of the brain responsible for learning and memory. What's more, those who painted pictures reported feeling less stress and depres-sion, and were found to be more psycho-logically resilient.

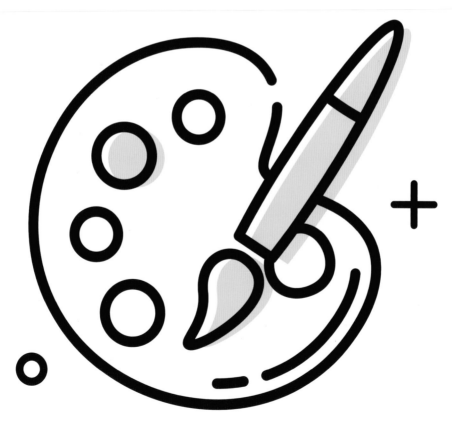

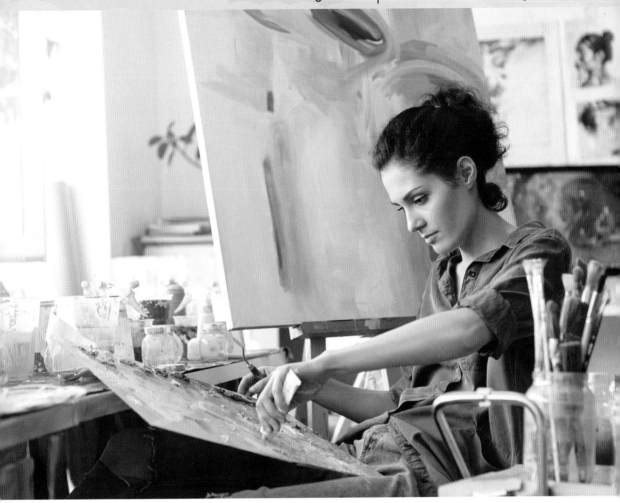

Another study found that people are more likely to remember information that they draw than information that they write or photograph. Study participants were given a list of 30 nouns and asked to write out half of them and draw the other half. When they were later asked to recall the words, the volunteers were able to remember twice as many of the drawn words as the written words.

Most interestingly, this result was the same for participants of all ages.

Don't worry if you've never been artistic; creative ability makes no difference with the benefits of painting. Pick up some supplies and create whatever comes to mind. Or, if you'd prefer a more guided experience, search for adult painting classes near your home.

o x + o x + o

35 Take Up Journaling

As moody teenagers, many of us would retreat to our bedrooms at the end of a day and dig out our hidden journals, beginning an entry with "Dear Diary" and filling pages with hopes and dreams. But there's no reason that journaling shouldn't continue into adulthood; in fact, a regular journaling practice not only helps you keep a record of important events in your life, but it is also a great way to keep your brain healthy.

With the proliferation of social media, a 24/7 news cycle, and hundreds of distracting television channels, it can be difficult to quiet our minds. Journaling provides a simple way to shut out the rest of the world and organize thoughts and ideas and make sense of what is often a chaotic life. And the benefits of this practice are numerous. Journaling helps you to examine your thoughts critically and logically, providing clarity while also prompting focus and organization. It also helps to reduce stress and anxiety, increase creativity, and serves as a reminder of past accomplishments and happy milestones.

Best of all, writing down experiences makes it easier to recall details later on, and expressive writing, such as journaling, improves working memory. But to get the most benefit, scientists recommend journaling at bedtime, which increases the chance of recalling the written information the next day. Researchers believe this is because the things we think about just before falling asleep are consolidated and cemented into our minds during slumber.

So if you think that keeping a diary is only for teenagers, think again!

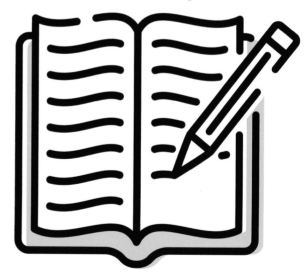

36 Read a Long Book

Many movies and television shows are based on books: *Gone With the Wind*, *Jurassic Park*, the *Lord of the Rings* trilogy, *Game of Thrones*.

But how many times have we heard someone say that the book was so much better than the movie? Well, according to scientists, reading that long book instead of watching the truncated movie version doesn't just provide you with a better story line and better developed characters, but it's also great for your brain!

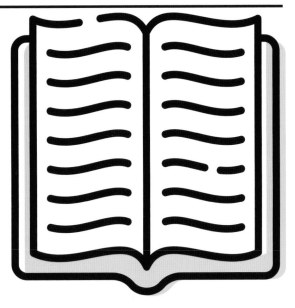

With our busy electronic lifestyles, many of us prefer the ease of logging on to our favorite news site to read about current events or relaxing in front of a Netflix show at the end of the day. But trying to read through an actual newspaper or spending time absorbed in a good book are better ways to engage our brains. Reading is a more neurobiologically complex process than looking at visual images, activating many parts of the brain at the same time. Concentration and a creative thought process are required to construct images in our minds of the words we read, and, since reading provides a way to pause and comprehend, the brain works harder than when we simply watch a movie or television show.

Studies show that reading improves connections between different areas of the brain, and the mental exercise it provides reduces the risk of dementia and Alzheimer's while protecting memory and thinking skills.

Read the book instead of seeing the movie. Not only will the story be more fulfilling, but you'll give your brain a boost, as well.

37 Keep Up With the News

When it comes to preventing memory loss, scientists have several concrete suggestions. Some of these seem to be a matter of common sense, such as engaging in exercise and eating a healthy diet. When your body is healthy, your brain has a greater chance of enjoying good health, too. Other suggestions include maintaining an active social life, getting quality sleep, and managing stress. All of these add up to a lifestyle that gives you the most benefit for your brain.

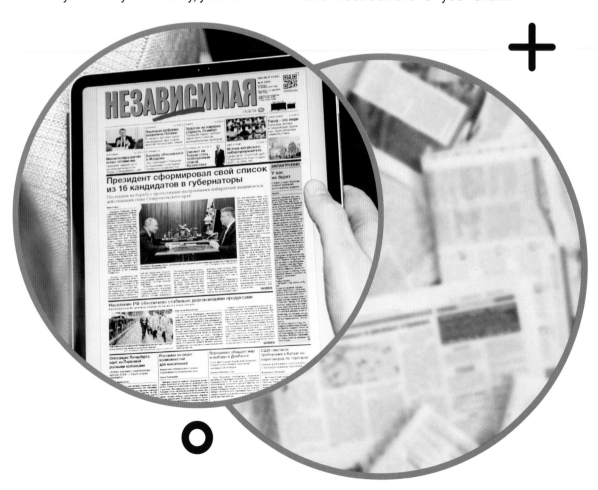

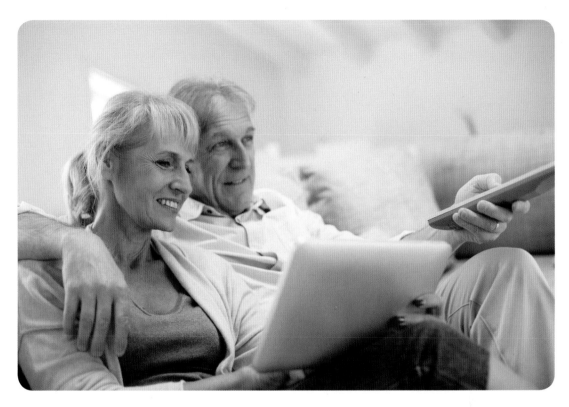

But one suggestion is even simpler than all the others: Keeping up with the news. Reading up on current events doesn't seem like an activity that would affect your brain, but it turns out that it's more beneficial than we realize. In fact, older adults who read the news on a regular basis are about 17 percent less likely to develop Alzheimer's than those who don't pay attention to current events.

Scientists believe this may be because reading about current events can often trigger memories and emotions in the brain, as well as providing it with new information. Since any kind of brain stimulation is beneficial for keeping it healthy, reading the news on a daily basis is an easy way to give it a bit of a workout.

No matter how old we are, our brains are capable of learning and forming connections between brain cells. Staying informed about what's going on in the world is one way to challenge the brain and protect it from decline.

38 Get Outside

After a day of working in an office, doing household chores, or just dealing with the usual stresses of life, we often feel as if we could use a "breath of fresh air." Although we sometimes use the phrase in a metaphorical way, getting outside into the fresh air—literally—may be just what we need to keep our brains happy and healthy.

In fact, some studies suggest that spending time outdoors is not only beneficial but may be necessary to maintain good health. Interacting with nature has been proven to reduce high blood pressure, improve mood, reduce anxiety, and provide an overall feeling of life satisfaction.

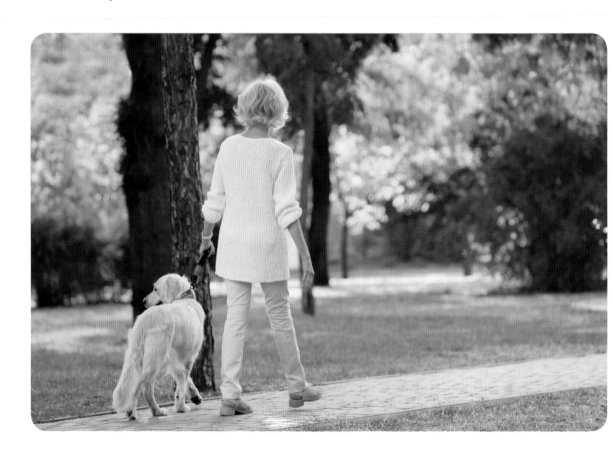

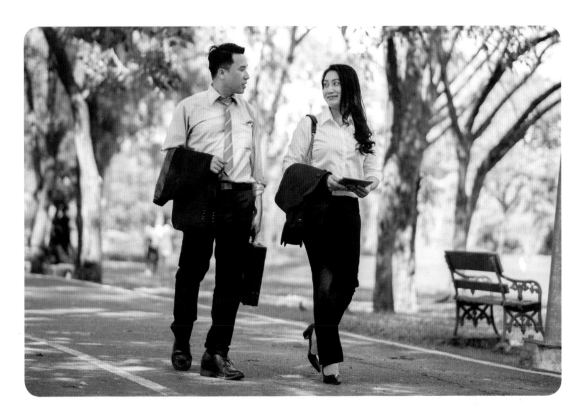

Walking through nature has also been shown to increase attention span, boost creativity, and improve short-term memory. In one study performed at the University of Michigan, volunteers were asked to either walk a route through downtown Ann Arbor or to take a detour through a botanical garden and arboretum. Afterwards, those who had taken the nature walk had improved their working memory by around 20 percent.

And it doesn't matter whether it's summer or winter, or if you're walking through a park or playing in the snow; any time spent outdoors will have an effect. So take a stroll through a forest, sled down a snowy hill, or simply sit on a park bench during your lunch hour. Any time spent in the great outdoors adds up to big brain benefits.

o x + o x + o

39 Do Things Out Loud

Do you ever find yourself talking out loud even if you're the only one in the room? Don't be embarrassed; in fact, keep it up! Talking out loud, even if you look a little silly while you're doing it, improves memory retention.

A recent study published in the aptly titled journal *Memory* asked volunteers to remember as many words as possible from a list of 160 nouns. Participants either read the words aloud, read them silently, or heard recordings of the words being read aloud. Two weeks later they were tested to determine how many words they could recall. Across the board, reading the words out loud helped the volunteers remember more words than any of the other scenarios.

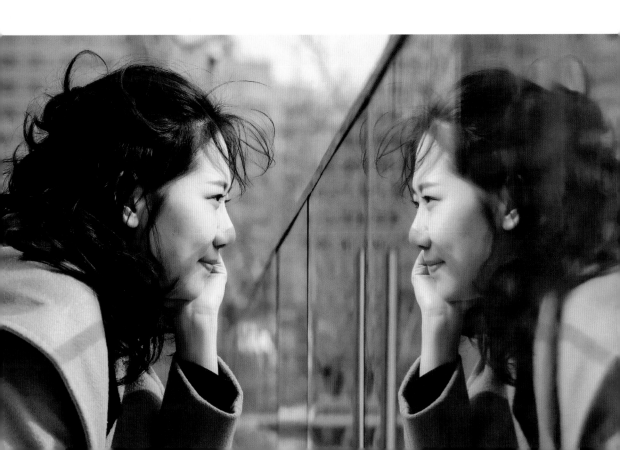

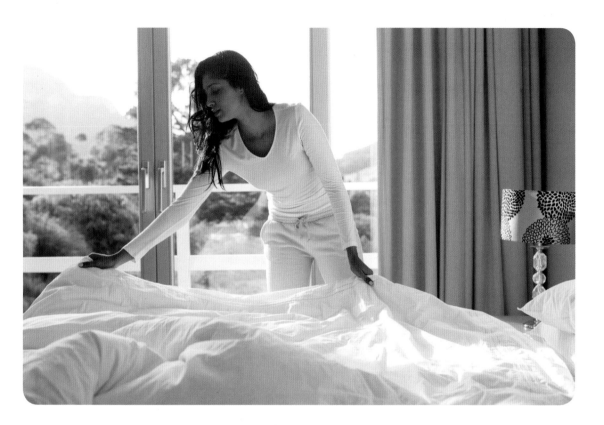

Scientists believe this is due to a phenomenon called the "production effect." When we say something aloud, it is turned into speech, which not only gives our brains the knowledge of producing that speech, but also the memory of hearing the speech. This one-two punch gives the spoken items a more significant distinction in our brains, translating to a greater chance of remembering them later. The distinction makes the spoken items stand out—similar to how we always remember events that are out of the ordinary, but are less likely to recall the boring minutes of life.

If you have some important information to remember, try talking about it out loud. You may look a little silly, but you'll leave your brain with a lasting impression!

o X + o X + o

40 Listen to Podcasts

Remember when television and radio were the only options for broadcast entertainment? You could watch a show on television, or listen to music or the news on the radio, but that was about it. And if you were away from home, your choices were even more limited.

But fast-forward to the twenty-first century, and our entertainment options are practically unlimited. We're not even bound by schedules anymore, with "on-demand" programing becoming more and more popular. And while there's plenty of "mindless" entertainment out there, we also have the opportunity to increase our knowledge and brainpower through podcasts.

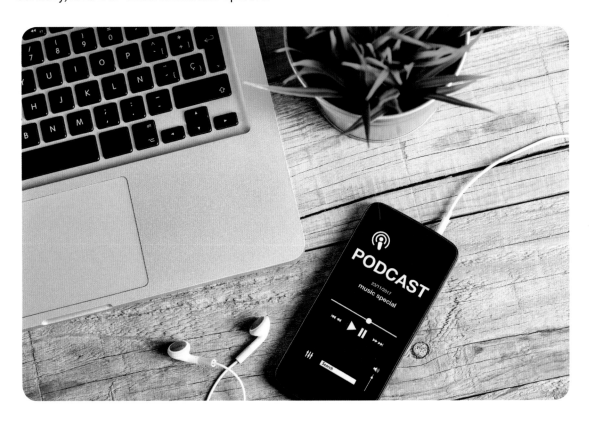

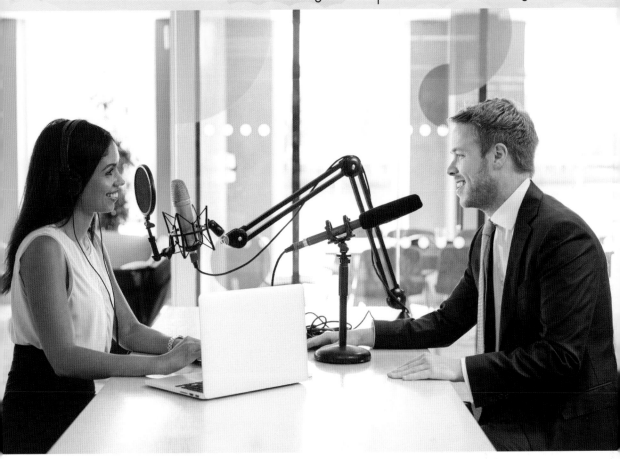

Podcasts are kind of like talk radio shows, but you can listen anytime and any place by downloading an app to your phone. And scientists have discovered that listening to podcasts engages your brain in an active way. Our brain needs to work hard to take in the audio content of a podcast and turn it into a sensory experience, activating not only the part of the brain that processes language but parts that correspond to the subject matter.

So to help activate your memory, download a free podcast app and start listening to some podcasts developed just for that reason.

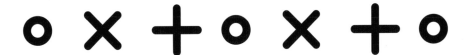

41 Remember Names

Most of us can remember faces quite easily, even if we've only seen them once or twice. But when it comes to attaching a name to that face, that's another matter entirely. We tend to remember faces more readily because it involves the process of recognition, whereas attaching a name to the face requires a process called recall. Recognition is much easier for the brain to accomplish, because recognition simply requires you to choose among a limited number of alternatives that are present in front of your eyes—sort of like a multiple-choice question. But to recall a name, the brain has to go digging for it, which is a much more complex process. Recall, then, is more like a fill-in-the-blank question.

The process of recall is generally easier if we have some retrieval cues that give the brain some direction. One way to do this is to associate an individual's name with another piece of information that you already know.

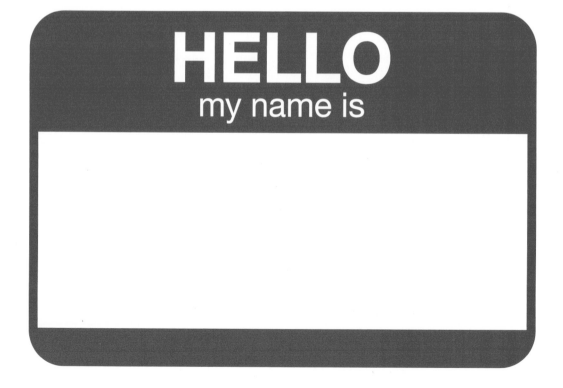

HELLO
my name is

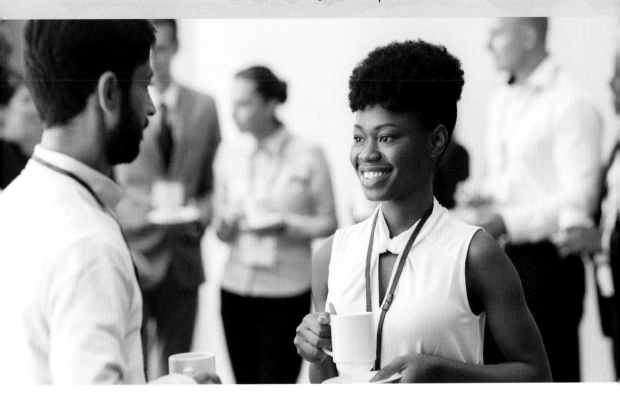

For example, when you first meet a person and hear their name, you might tell yourself that this person has the same name as your mother-in-law or the same name as your favorite baseball player.

You can also use the verbal technique to help implant a person's name in your memory when you first meet them. To do this, simply:

1. Register the person's name: Pay attention to it as it is said!

2. Repeat the person's name to yourself.

3. Comment on the name.

4. Use the person's name out loud as soon as possible.

42 Organize Your Life

It should come as no surprise that disorganization can be bad for our brains. After all, if we walk into a room to look for our keys and end up getting distracted by clutter, we're apt to forget why we entered the room in the first place!

Add in our daily barrage of emails and text messages, plus the websites and other media we're exposed to, and it's no wonder we can't always remember everything we see, hear, or read.

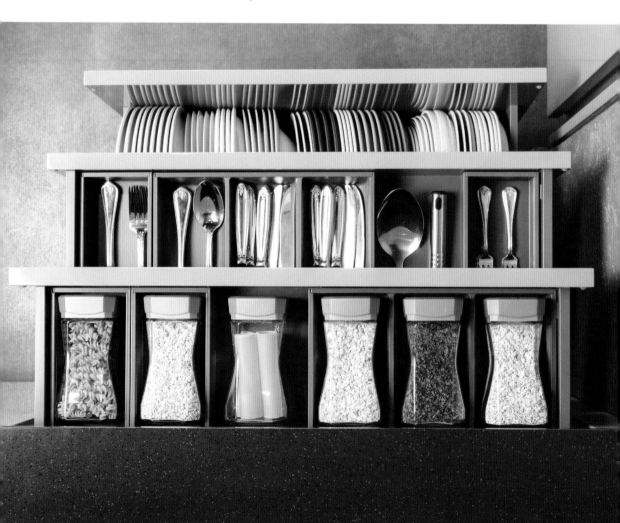

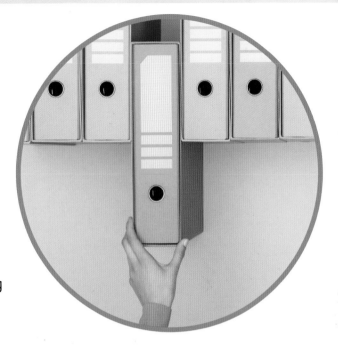

Some scientists like to think of working memory as a notepad that keeps track of items in our brain. The things we remember are added to the notepad and then stored in the brain for later retrieval. But clutter and an avalanche of information make it much more difficult to form coherent items for the notepad.

So how do we counteract all the clutter? Organize, of course! Experts recommend several strategies for clearing away distractions and giving working memory a hand:

- Make sure to place keys, sunglasses, and other necessary items in the same place every day. When items have a "home," they are easier to remember.

- Always write down appointments on a calendar and tasks on a to-do list.

- Keep a small notebook and pen handy to immediately write down important thoughts throughout the day.

- Make use of the "bookmarks" feature on your web browser to keep all of your favorite websites handy.

Clearing away physical clutter—or "visual noise"—is helpful, as well. The more you simplify and minimize distractions, the better working memory will function.

43 Be Busy

As we get older, many of us look forward to retirement, a time when we can finally tackle some home improvement projects, travel the world, or simply do nothing at all. But it turns out that doing nothing may be the worst choice when it comes to keeping your brain healthy.

Studies have shown that keeping a busy schedule as you get older has just as many brain benefits as engaging in mentally challenging activities like puzzles or crafting. It seems that when the mind is kept busy, it forces the brain to learn and grow.

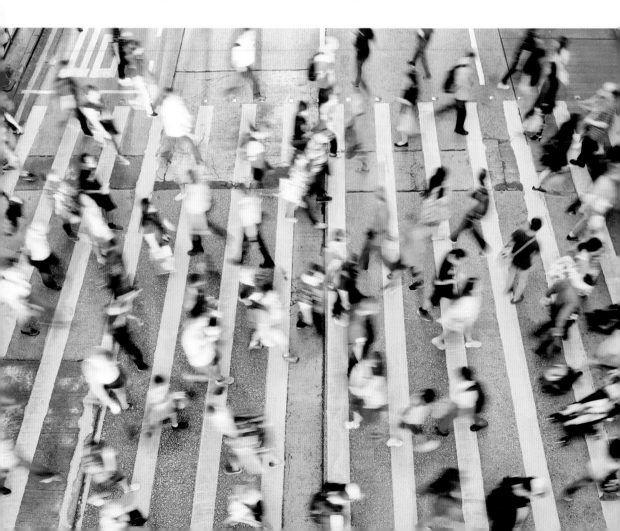

A recent study followed a group of 300 people between ages 50 to 89. Researchers tested the group on their cognition skills at the beginning of the study and again four years later. Researchers discovered that those who reported being busiest tested highest on processing speed, working memory, episodic memory, reasoning, and knowledge.

Scientists theorize that this occurs because keeping busy exposes you to new situations, opportunities, and people, which gives the brain a chance to continually process unfamiliar information. This, in turn, keeps neurons in the hippocampus firing, leading to better memory and a quicker thought process.

There is one caveat, though: Experts warn against overcommitting and staying busy to the point of feeling stressed and anxious. But keeping your calendar filled with activities that are fun, fulfilling, and meaningful—while adding in some time to relax and recharge, as well—can help your brain stay sharp.

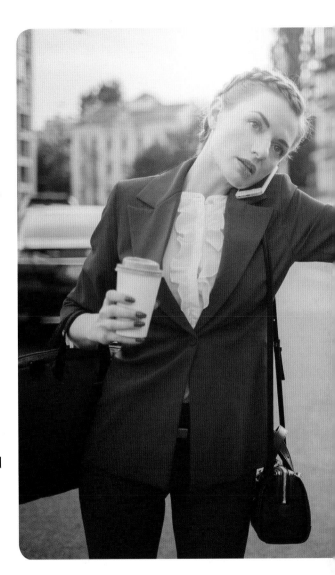

o x + o x + o

44 Break Up Your Routine

There's something to be said for having a routine. A daily routine makes it easy to remember everything that needs to be done, helps reduce stress levels, and gives us a way to cultivate healthy habits. But did you know that breaking your routine can offer its own benefits? It may seem a bit scary or unsettling, but shaking things up once in a while can be a great way to give your brain a workout.

When we follow a routine day after day, we're essentially functioning on "auto-pilot." This means that our brain follows the same neural pathways over and over, free of challenges or unexpected information. It doesn't need to work very hard to pour the same bowl of cereal, walk to the same coffee shop, drive to the same office, or head to the same gym every single day. In order to give your brain some extra exercise, try changing things up and varying your routine.

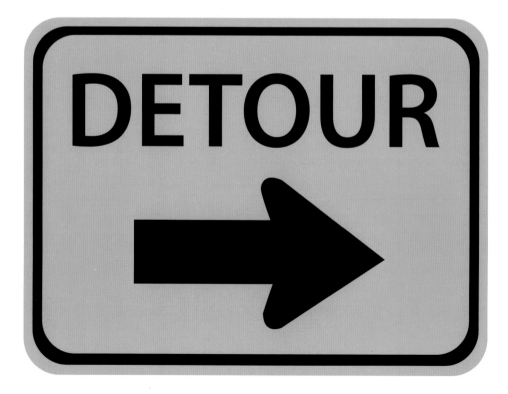

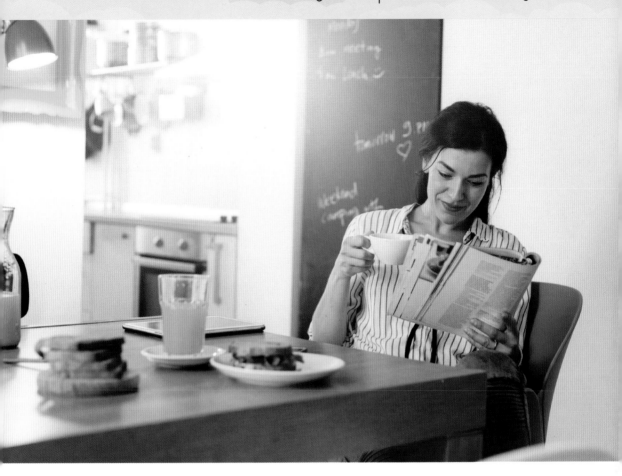

The changes don't need to be major. For instance, you may not be able to avoid going to the office every day, but try taking a different route to get there. Along the way, stop at a different coffee shop and meet some new people. These small tweaks are surprisingly impactful, as they force the brain to process new scenarios.

You can break up your routine in more significant ways by learning some new skills, joining a club, or finding a new hobby. Remember, the brain thrives on change, so don't be afraid to switch things up!

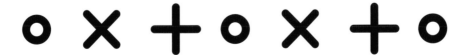

45 Take a Mental Timeout

How many times have you found yourself completely stumped by a problem to the point you can't even stand to think about it anymore? Maybe you take a break—like a walk, a chat with a friend, or a trip to a coffee shop—and when you return to the problem, suddenly the answer is apparent! This phenomenon demonstrates the amazing power of taking a mental timeout.

And the benefits don't stop at problem-solving skills. Taking breaks can also help to strengthen memories, especially of information recently learned. A study performed at New York University's Center for Neural Science used functional magnetic resonance imaging (fMRI) to monitor the activity in the brains of volunteers, who were shown pairs of images and then allowed a mental timeout.

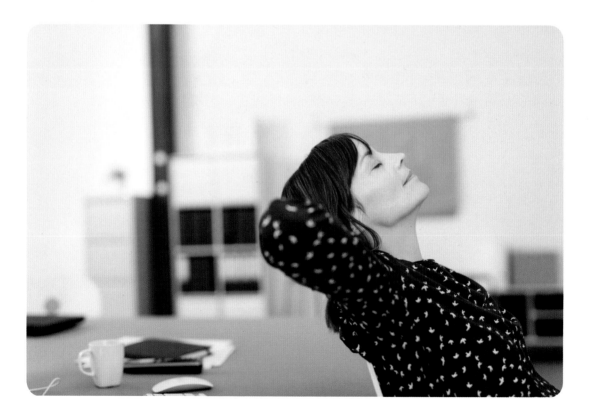

The participants were not informed that they would later be tested on their memory; researchers simply told them to think about whatever they wanted. Yet when reviewing the fMRIs, the researchers noticed a strong connection between the part of the brain that was active when the volunteers first looked at the pictures, and the hippocampus when the participants were taking a break. What's more, this connection seemed to make it easier for the volunteers to later recall the images they'd previously seen.

The bottom line seems to be that taking mental breaks helps the brain form memories; breaks give the brain time to review and instill the information.

So don't feel guilty about taking an occasional coffee break. You're giving your brain just what it needs!

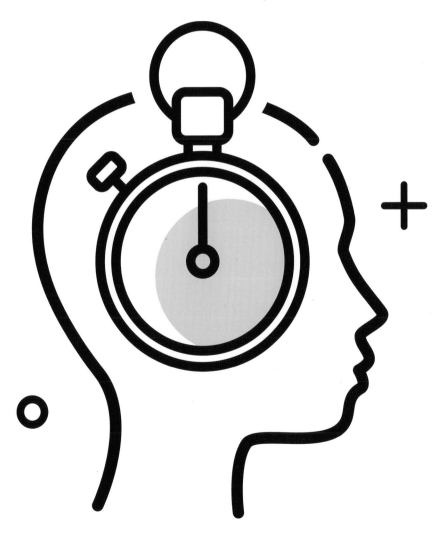

46 Don't Procrastinate

Many of us are great procrastinators. We wonder why we should doing something today when we can do it tomorrow. If you're a procrastinator, you can't afford to put off reading this section. Putting work, projects, or tasks off almost always has bad consequences, one of which is disturbed sleep. Getting your work done can be seen as another way of managing your stress. You can choose to put your time and energy into accomplishing what is before you and reap the benefits or put it off and worry about it. Tasks left undone can even intrude into your dreams at night and, in extreme cases, lead to nightmares.

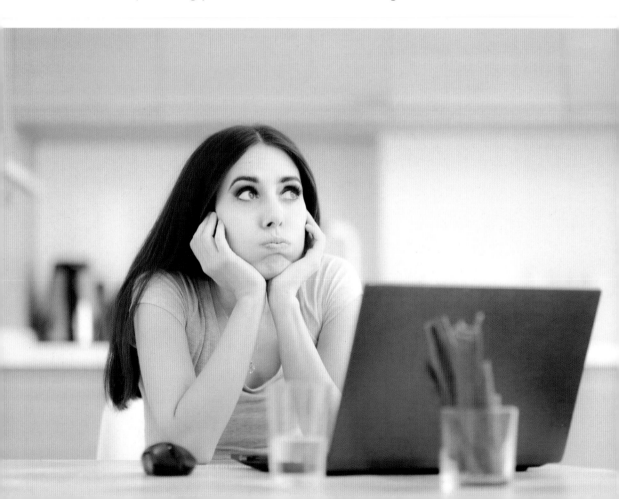

Avoiding procrastination takes some discipline. There are certain techniques, however, that can help:

• Make a "to-do" list for the day. Then rank your list from most to least important. Start with the most important and work your way through. If unexpected circumstances limit what you can accomplish that day, you will have put your limited time and energy toward the most important tasks. And this will leave you with a sense of accomplishment.

• Keep promises to do tasks on time. Make schedules and stick with them. When promised work is late, it only becomes more difficult to face as time goes by.

• Finish what you start. Leaving projects half done is sometimes worse than not starting them at all. An incomplete job will occupy your mind and make relaxing difficult. Also, work that is partly done robs you of the satisfaction that comes with closure.

• Learn to say "no." Sometimes we procrastinate because we feel overwhelmed by all of our commitments. Still, we continue to volunteer for tasks or projects because we don't want to tell someone "no." To combat this habit, make an effort to look realistically at your schedule and responsibilities before you commit to optional activities.

47 Phone a Friend

As we get older and life changes, it can be difficult to maintain strong friendships. We have kids, our friends have kids, everyone has a busy schedule, and it's often hard to connect in a meaningful way. Add in work responsibilities, relocations, and other major life upsets, and friendships often take a backseat to the many duties we handle on a daily basis.

Although it can take some effort, maintaining the bond you have with your bestie is not only great for your social life, but it can help to keep your brain young, too. Studies show that friendship can be just as beneficial as diet and exercise for keeping the brain healthy, and it might even be more beneficial than spending time with our own families!

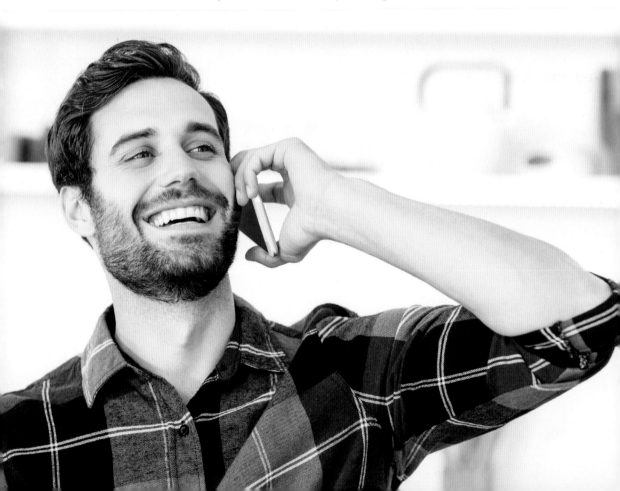

One study, which researched the lives of people over the age of 80, found that those who had close, trusting relationships with friends were more likely to have impressive memory and cognitive skills and a lower risk of cognitive decline, impairment, and dementia.

There's another interesting benefit to having a friend on speed dial, and it's something called "memory extension." This is the idea that some of the information we need may not be constantly stored in our own brains, but rather in other locations. Take photos, for instance. We may not always remember every minute of a favorite vacation, but by

looking at a photo, those memories can be retrieved.

In the same way, phoning a friend may help you both recall memories and events from your past, while giving you both a healthy brain boost. So make the effort to stay connected!

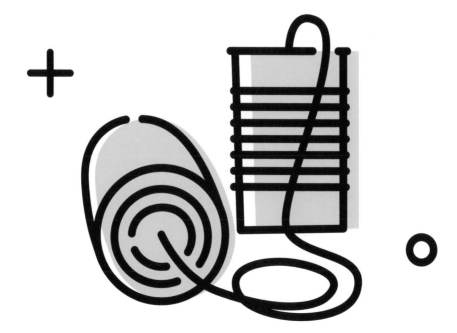

48 Track Down Old Friends

Staying in touch with a best friend is definitely a boon for your brain. But what about friends we haven't seen in years or even decades? It turns out that reconnecting with old friends can bring some unexpected benefits, even if you haven't spoken a word to each other in a long time.

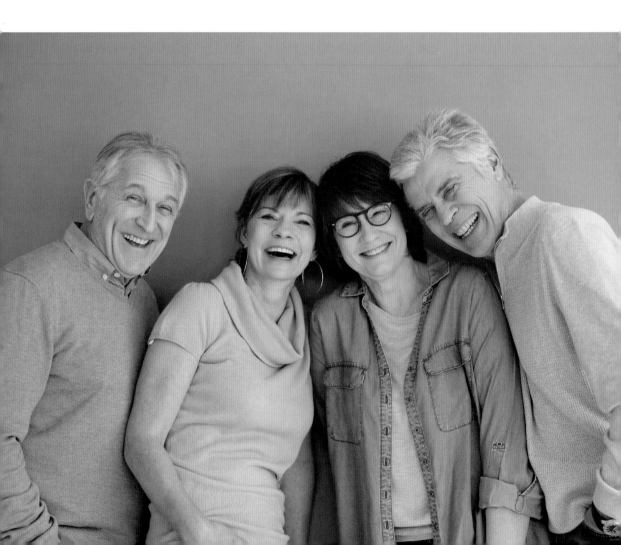

Many of us will find ourselves feeling lonely at one time or another during our lives. Moving to a new city or retiring from an office job can leave us feeling isolated and cut off from the world. And in our online age, everything from banking to grocery shopping can be done behind a computer screen, giving us even fewer reasons to interact with people. But fortunately, the same technology that isolates us can be used to connect us, as well.

It's easier than ever to find old friends merely by searching online. And making those reconnections can be hugely beneficial, especially if you feel isolated or doubt your own social skills. Renewing an old friendship helps us to feel less anxious and insecure about these things.

But even more than that, talking with old friends gives us a reminder of things past. You and your friend share memories that go back decades; even if you haven't spoken in years, those memories can resurface, giving you both a connection to your personal history. And maintaining your rekindled relationship can decrease your risk for dementia, depression, and heart disease. It's a worthwhile endeavor to take a chance and find some long-lost friends.

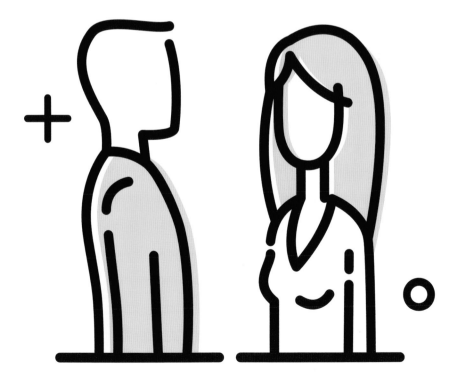

49 Join a Club

Did you have a clubhouse when you were a child (maybe complete with a "keep out" sign)? Well, clubs aren't just for kids. Adults have some great options when it comes to joining clubs, and not only do they eschew the "keep out" signs, but they provide plenty of healthy brain benefits, too!

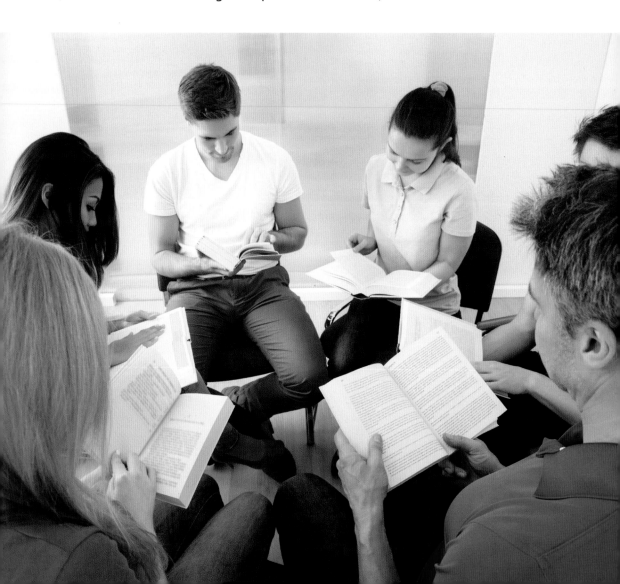

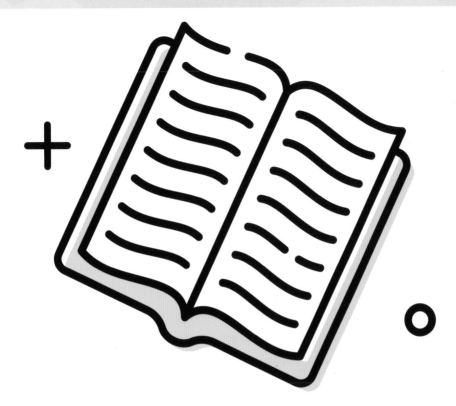

Joining a club may be especially beneficial for older adults, as loneliness and isolation become a risk as we get older. Sometimes this isolation is deliberate. A survey conducted by AARP found that 87 percent of people over the age of 65 would prefer to stay in their current home indefinitely, even after losing a spouse. Although this provides a sense of comfort and familiarity, it can also result in a feeling of being cut off from the world. And with approximately 12.5 million older Americans living alone, finding ways to socialize can be extremely important.

Studies have shown that isolation can be detrimental to health, increasing the possibility of cognitive decline, depression, and even infections. But socializing as we age has the opposite effect, lowering the risk of dementia, decreasing depression, and strengthening the immune system. Joining a club can be the perfect way to keep some socialization in your life, even if you prefer to live alone.

50 Try Karaoke

In the early 1970s, the first karaoke machine was created in Japan, allowing amateur singers to sing along to recorded instrumental music. Karaoke—a blend of the Japanese words kara (meaning "empty") and a shortened form of okesutora (meaning "orchestra")—was first marketed to bars and hotels, and it provided patrons with gimmicky entertainment that enticed them to stay a little longer and order a few more drinks.

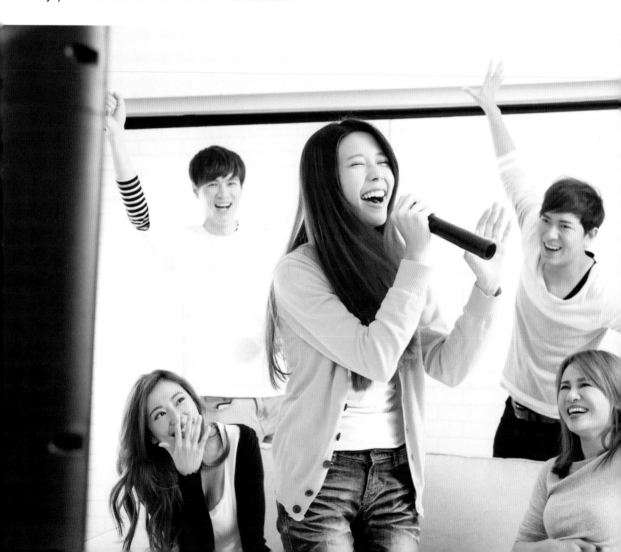

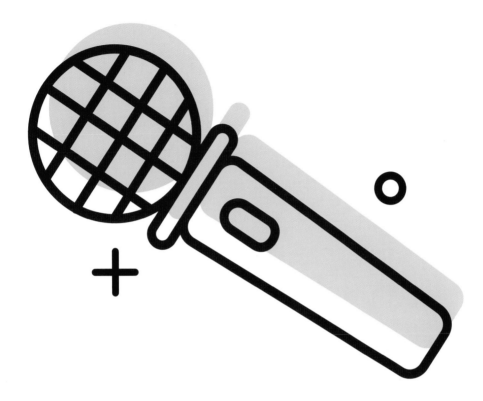

Karaoke itself later became a main attraction, and the Japanese fad took off in other parts of the world. Today, it's easy to find a bar, restaurant, or entertainment facility that features karaoke in any big city in the country. You can even buy or rent your own machine and invite friends and family to a karaoke night!

And surprisingly, this musical craze may offer some benefits to its performers, besides giving you the opportunity to showcase your talent. Karaoke allows you to socialize, relieve stress, and build your confidence. Even better, the activity gives your brain a workout, for singing requires following a rhythm, melody, and lyrics. If you know the song, your brain automatically works to access your memories about it, and if you don't know it, the lyrics are implanted in your memory as soon as you sing.

The next time you hear someone singing off-key karaoke, be sure to give them a hand anyway. In fact, do your brain a favor and join in!

51 Care for Grandkids

Some people say that grandkids are the best part of growing older. Not only do you get to witness your own children becoming parents, but you also get to experience all of the love and fun that goes along with raising kids—without all the responsibility! Of course, you may be called up to step in and change a diaper or two on those occasions when the kids need a babysitter. And if the chance arises, you should definitely jump at it; taking care of grandkids is greatly beneficial for your brain.

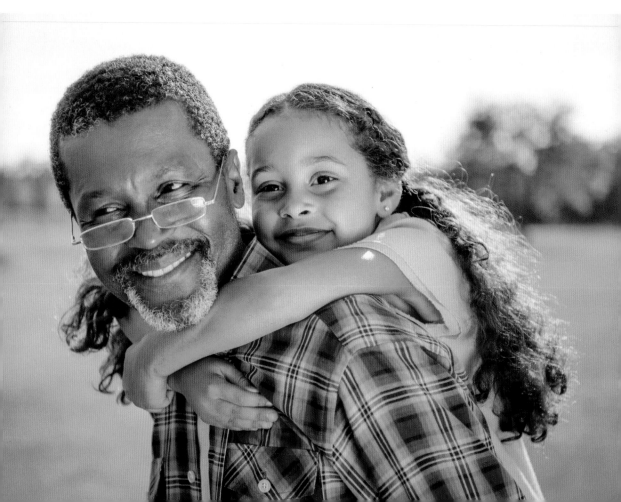

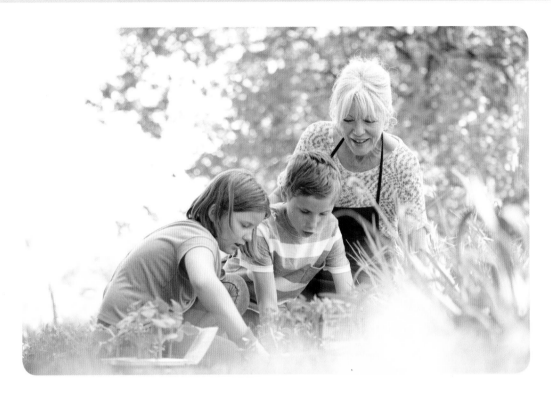

Studies have found that grandparents who regularly care for their grandchildren exhibit better working memory and a lower risk of depression and Alzheimer's. A strong bond between grandparents and grandchildren was also shown to lessen the risk of depression. A study performed by Boston College followed 376 grandparents and their grandchildren over the course of 19 years, and it discovered that those who shared the closest bonds were the least likely to suffer from depression—grandparent and grandchild alike.

Scientists believe that the positive effect of caring for grandchildren stems from the social interaction of being around family. Preventing social isolation can be crucial for maintaining good health as we age. What better way to spend time than with grandkids?

While the benefits of babysitting are many, experts warn that there can be too much of a good thing: Those who felt worn out or overextended by their babysitting duties were more likely to score negatively on cognitive tests, due to stress and fatigue. So be sure to balance the responsibility with plenty of fun; after all, that's the best part of being a grandparent!

52 Get a Pet

Everyone knows that dogs are "man's best friend." But whether you're a dog person or a cat person, having a furry companion is beneficial for reasons beyond friendship. In fact, having a pet provides a unique way to tick off many of the boxes on the "healthy brain" checklist.

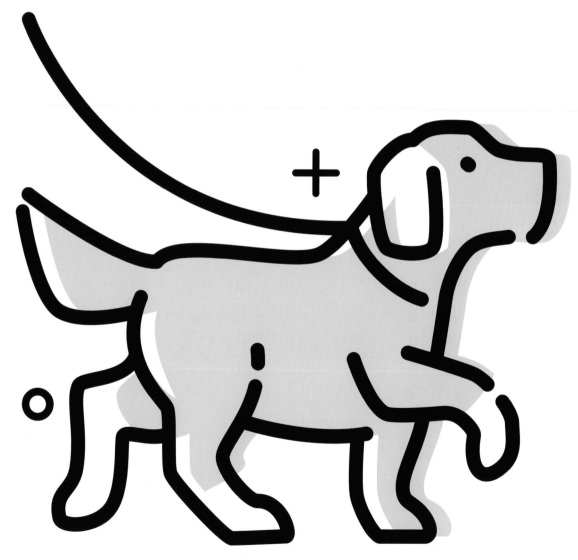

For instance, having a dog or cat provides an automatic companion at anytime, helping to stave off loneliness and the depression that can accompany it. Bonding with an animal can fill the void that comes with living alone. They also provide an excuse to exercise; dogs require daily walks or games of fetch, and even cats benefit from games with string or other toys.

Having a pet—especially one who enjoys daily walks—also gives you an excuse to socialize. A walk through the park can introduce you to other pet owners, but even regular visits to the vet, pet stores, or groomers gives pet owners a reason to stay connected to people. Pets also give us a sense of purpose.

Countless studies have proven the benefits of pet ownership, demonstrating that older adults who own pets have lower blood pressure and a lower risk of heart disease than those who don't own pets.

Keeping blood pressure under control and getting regular exercise are two of the best preventive measures you can take to prevent dementia and Alzheimer's disease. Having a best friend to help keep you accountable is just icing on the cake!

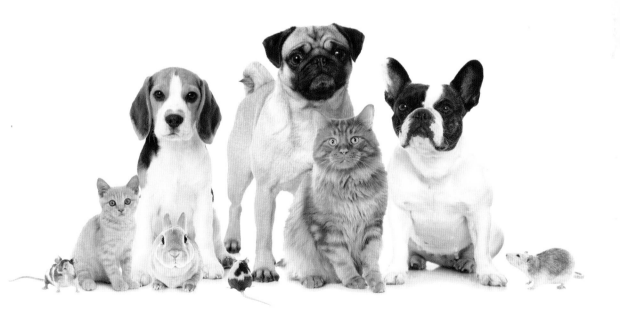

53 Purchase a Fish Tank or Terrarium

If your doctor's or dentist's office has a fish tank in the waiting room, chances are it's not just for decoration. Watching fish swim has a soothing, relaxing effect, and it helps to reduce anxiety and heart rate. Staring at a fish tank for as little as five minutes can result in an almost hypnotic effect, helping us to calm down before that dreaded root canal. But why wait until you visit a doctor? Adding a fish tank to your home lets you enjoy its benefits anytime.

Studies have shown that gazing at fish in an aquarium can decrease heart rate by more than 7 percent. There is even evidence that watching fish swim decreases feelings of pain. In fact, this is one of the reasons aquariums are so prevalent in medical offices. Research has found that dental patients who watch fish in an aquarium before their appointment experience less pain during treatment and require less pain medication during recovery. No wonder fish tanks are so common at the dentist!

Fish tanks are also used as therapy for those suffering from Alzheimer's disease. Aquariums—especially those with brightly colored fish—have been shown to calm patients and reduce aggressiveness. Those exposed to aquariums were also found to have better short-term memory and required less medication.

The best part about this fishy brain boost is that you don't need a huge aquarium to reap the benefits. Any size aquarium, large or small, will do. Before choosing fish for an aquarium, be sure to visit a local pet store and ask which fish are best for its size.

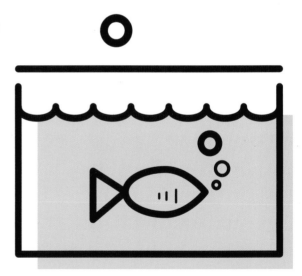

54   Volunteer

Retiring after a long career can bring some great new opportunities into your life. You have time to travel, explore new hobbies, and visit family. But sometimes, the end of a career can mean fewer chances to socialize, leading to feelings of isolation or loneliness. Fortunately, one of the best ways to break out of isolation is not only good for you, but good for others, as well: volunteering.

Recent studies have shown all kinds of benefits for older adults who volunteer. Two of these studies were performed in 2015 by the Corporation for National and Community Service (CNCS), which discovered that 70 percent of retired individuals who volunteered reported a decrease in feelings of depression, and 67 percent said they had gained more social connections.

In addition to preventing depression and increasing social activity, volunteering helps to keep the brain active, giving it new and meaningful information to process, which helps to protect memory and lowers the risk of dementia. Volunteering also provides an opportunity to stay active, which is one of the most important steps you can take to keep your brain healthy.

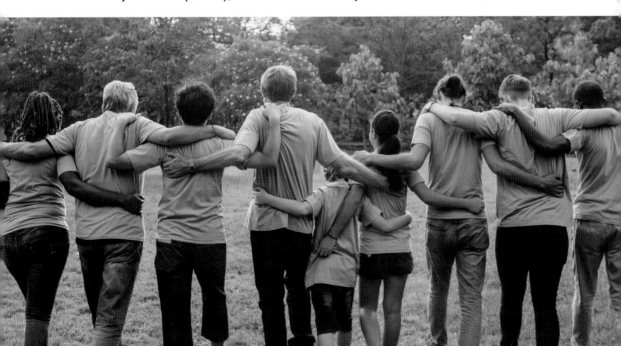

55 Go Fishing or Hunting

We've all seen the scenario play out on television or in a movie: Overwhelmed with work and responsibilities, a character sneaks away from urban civilization and heads out to the country to fish in a lake or hunt in the woods (perhaps giving the "I'm sick in bed" excuse). Of course, the charade is inevitably discovered, usually with hilarious consequences. But it's no joke that fishing and hunting can actually be good for you!

In fact, there are so many health benefits associated with these activities that you shouldn't feel guilty about taking a day to yourself once in a while to head into the great outdoors. Just being outside has been proven to provide the brain with a boost, as we remove ourselves from the stress of our usual schedules, deadlines, and appointments and connect with nature.

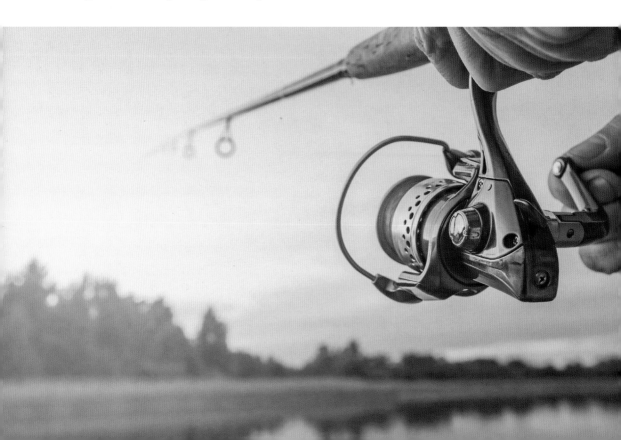

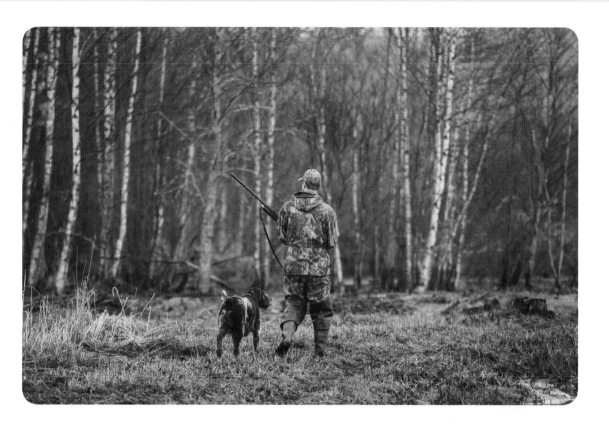

And while fishing and hunting come with the obvious benefit of exercise—which has been shown to increase the size of the hippocampus and preserve memory function—the activities are also surprisingly mentally challenging. To succeed at fishing or hunting, one must tackle all kinds of problems that might arise, and seek out logical and creative solutions. Many experienced fishers and hunters believe that the activities are 90 percent mental, making these sports not only a good workout for your body but for your mind, too.

Fishing and hunting provide a perfect opportunity to socialize, whether it be with friends, family, or co-workers. And perhaps best of all, at the end of the day, you can sit down to a nutritious meal that you provided for yourself!

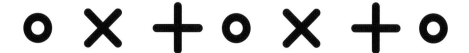

56 Get Political

Politics can be a nasty business. Watching candidates spar during debates or attack each other on social media is often disheartening. And the arguments that erupt between advocates of different issues can be enough to make us want to stop reading the news and just escape to a tropical island. So it would seem that there is no way the polarizing affair that is politics could possibly be good for us, right?

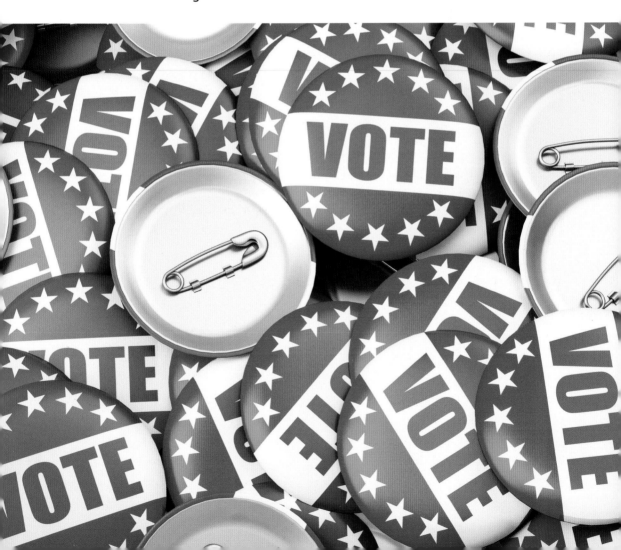

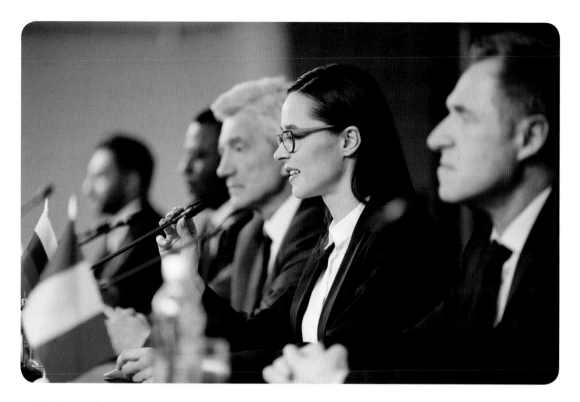

Well, surprisingly, participating in civic affairs—such as voting, volunteering for a campaign, or working on a community project—has been shown to produce healthy benefits. For one, participating in politics provides you with "social capital," which is the benefit of having shared group resources. As you socialize with like-minded individuals who are working toward a common goal, you may have the opportunity to meet their friends, and friends of friends. In other words, your social circle is automatically expanded, preventing the loneliness and isolation that can be so damaging as we age.

What's more, voting or helping others register to vote has been shown to improve health. A 2015 study that looked at 44 countries around the globe (including the U.S.) found that voters reported better overall health than non-voters. And volunteering in any capacity has been shown to be especially beneficial for older adults, decreasing the risk of cognitive impairment. So don't let political bickering deter you—contact one of your local candidates and ask how you can get involved.

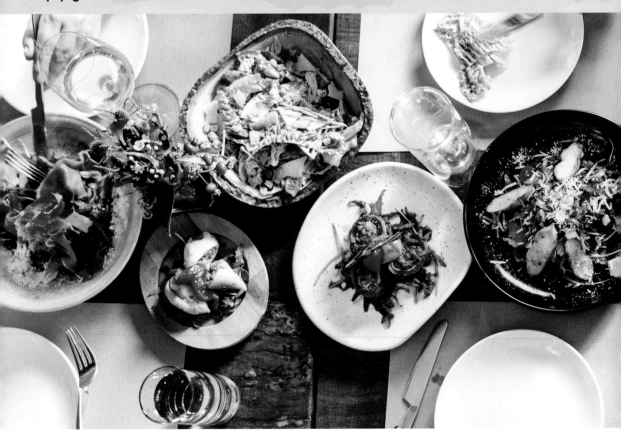

57 Visit New Restaurants

When we think about keeping our brains healthy, the first things that come to mind are probably puzzles, games, or other mental exercises. And learning new things is undoubtedly one of the best things we can do to keep our brain "on its toes." But remember, our brains control everything about us, from the way we think to the way we perceive sight and sound to the taste of the foods we eat.

o × + o × + o

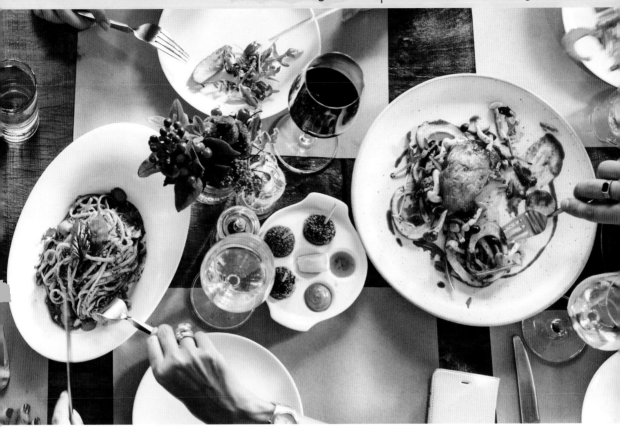

In fact, memories of food can be particularly strong. We all know of a certain food or candy with a taste that can transport us back to a moment in time. Maybe it's your grandmother's apple pie recipe, or a candy bar you used to buy at the corner store with your friends, or the stuffing your mom made for Thanksgiving every year. Food memories activate all of our senses, making them more powerful than most memories.

So what better way to give your brain a new kind of "workout" than to try new foods at new restaurants? It's easy to get into a restaurant rut, as we visit the same eateries over and over; but the novelty of trying something new is associated with the part of our brain that controls learning and memory. Just by trying a new restaurant, we fire up these areas of the brain and keep our memory working hard.

But here comes the best part: tasting new foods challenges all of your senses, giving the brain an extra (and delicious!) boost. Be mindful as you eat, and try to identify each ingredient in the new dishes you try. This keeps your taste buds—and your brain—guessing.

58 Go Camping

Most days, the average American spends around 10 hours indoors, staring at computer screens, televisions, or smartphones; but we spend less than 30 minutes a day outdoors. And that's a shame, because getting into nature is one of the best ways to not only give our brains a break from the cacophony of electronic devices, but it also strengthens our thinking skills and memory recall.

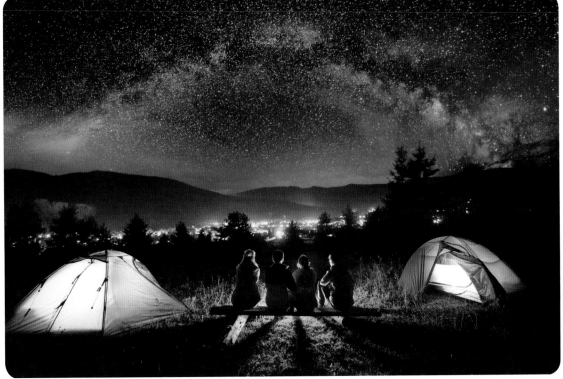

While simply taking a walk outdoors during your lunch hour can provide a nice respite for your brain, sometimes a longer break is in order. If short bursts of nature are good, how about an entire day (or weekend) in the fresh air? Camping can be a great way to reconnect with nature and with family or friends, and it provides a recharge for technology-addled brains.

Studies show that while short-term exposure to nature certainly helps decrease stress and improve memory, longer stays outdoors are even better. Research has shown that after three days of camping, the brain "resets" itself, resulting in increased productivity, better memory, and lower stress levels.

In addition to the restful benefits, camping provides other scenarios proven to give the brain a workout, including socialization and exercise. Plus, figuring out how to set up a tent, build a fire, or catch fish for dinner immerse you in new challenges that keep the brain working hard.

59 Take a Trip to the Zoo

Visit any zoo in the country and invariably you'll see children excitedly pointing and staring at their favorite animals. Groups of kids on field trips gather around lions and elephants as zookeepers offer facts and anecdotes about these creatures. It would be easy to think that zoos are only for children; but adults can benefit from them as well!

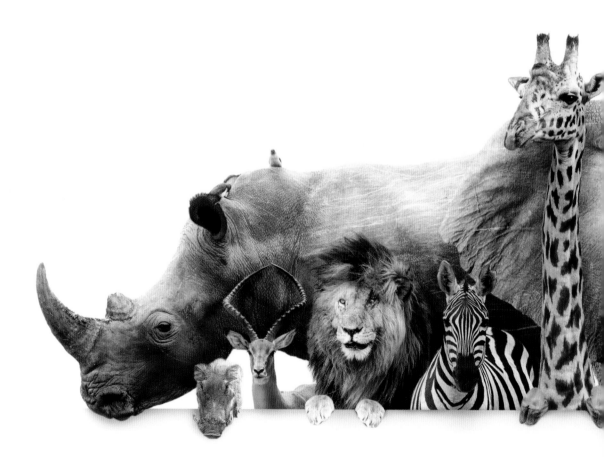

For starters, zoos provide an easy way to spend a few hours—or an entire day—surrounded by nature and a plethora of different animals, birds, fish, and vegetation. According to scientists, spending time with animals helps to lower blood pressure and increase feelings of happiness in people of all ages. And exposure to nature is one of the best ways to lower heart rate, reduce stress, and recharge the brain. A zoo provides a convenient way to surround yourself with the natural world (with the added bonus of benches and refreshment stands not found in nature!).

Zoos are often large, spread out over acres of land, giving you a perfect opportunity to exercise while taking in the wild sights. And of course, getting out and about is important, especially for older adults who are living alone. A trip to the zoo gives you an excuse to spend time with the grandkids or even just other adults.

Finally, the fascinating, unique world created by a zoo gives the brain a new and interesting experience to process, and it may even unlock hidden childhood memories, even in those who suffer from dementia. Taking a trip on the wild side may be just what your brain needs!

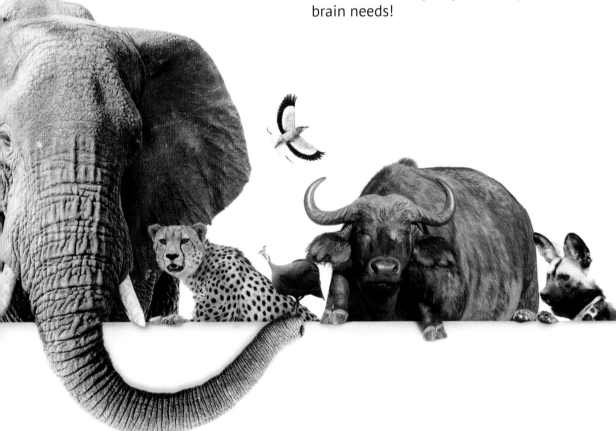

60 Throw a Party

After a week of work obligations and family responsibilities, sometimes we feel like letting off a little steam. And it turns out, throwing a party can actually be a healthy way to do just that. Parties may get a bad rap at times, since they often feature copious amounts of unhealthy food or alcohol; but studies show that having fun—in a responsible way—is good for us.

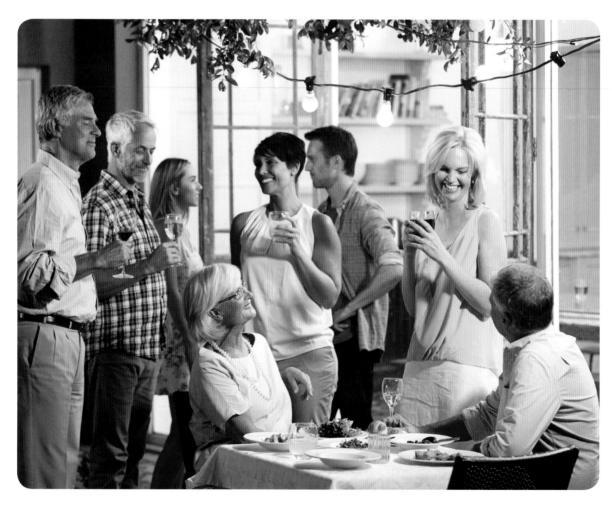

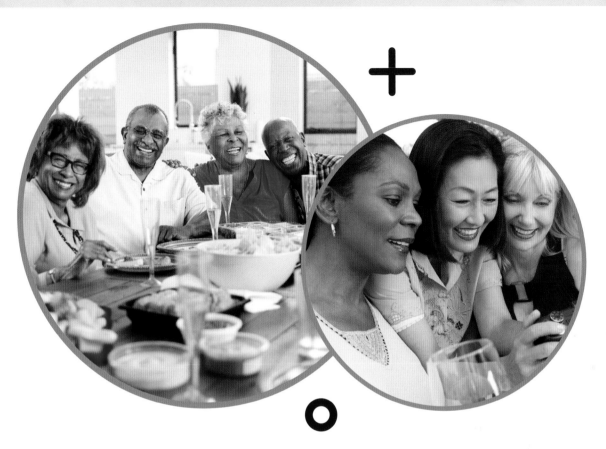

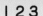

The benefits of throwing a party are numerous. Celebrating, even if it's just the end of a work week, gives us a sense of gratitude and reminds us of the positive things we have in our lives. Studies show that people who feel grateful also feel less stress and anxiety, have more energy, and enjoy better overall health than their pessimistic counterparts.

Having fun benefits us in other ways, too. It can relieve stress, improve brain function, and boost creativity. Parties promote socialization with friends and family, a crucial activity that has been shown to be vitally important for staving off dementia as we age.

Surprisingly, research is showing that even drinking alcohol can be good for the brain. One study discovered that low levels of alcohol—no more than a drink or two a day—decreases inflammation and eliminates proteins associated with Alzheimer's disease. So eat, drink, and be merry (in moderation). Your brain will be happier and healthier!

61 Go On a Scavenger Hunt

Most of us probably participated in a scavenger hunt or two when we were kids. Deciphering clues and searching for hidden treasures are fun ways to prevent boredom and spend time with friends. But like so many scenarios from childhood, scavenger hunts aren't just for kids anymore. In fact, scavenger hunts, including "geocaching"—in which participants use a GPS to find items hidden all over the world—are gaining popularity among adults.

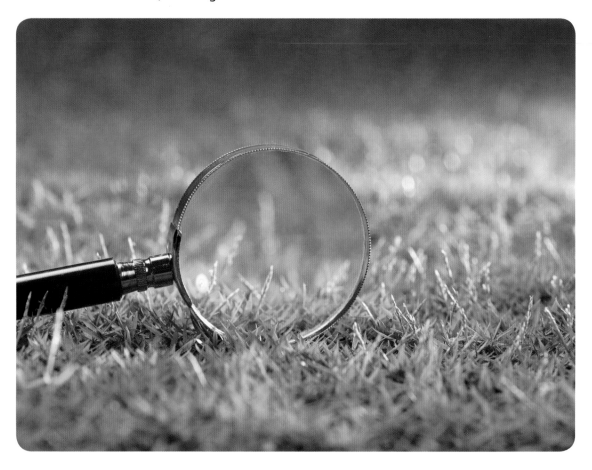

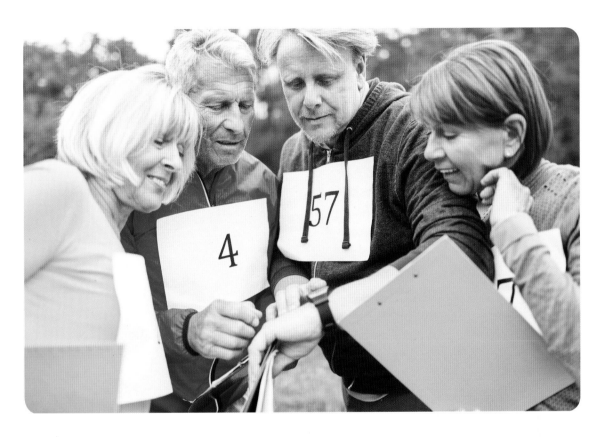

And there's good reason for this. It turns out that scavenger hunts are not only fun, but they come with all kinds of health benefits, too. Hunting for clues, "treasure," situations, or items requires a lot of exercise, as participants walk and travel from point A to point B. And if your scavenger hunt is set up as a race between different teams, the faster the better! What's more, a scavenger hunt encourages social interaction, not only between players on a team, but with people you encounter along the way.

Perhaps best of all, these games increase memory function as you navigate your way through the hunt. Using navigational skills and reading maps engages the brain, forcing it to tap into previously stored knowledge in the hippocampus, and solving puzzles or seeking solutions gives the brain a workout.

62 Make a Video

Have you ever been asked to pick up an item at the store, only to forget about it five minutes later? Or what about meeting someone new for the first time, and forgetting their name immediately after they speak it? You're not alone. In fact, it's quite common for the things we hear to be quickly forgotten. This is because our brain stores audio information in a more temporary way than other kinds of information, such as pictures or video.

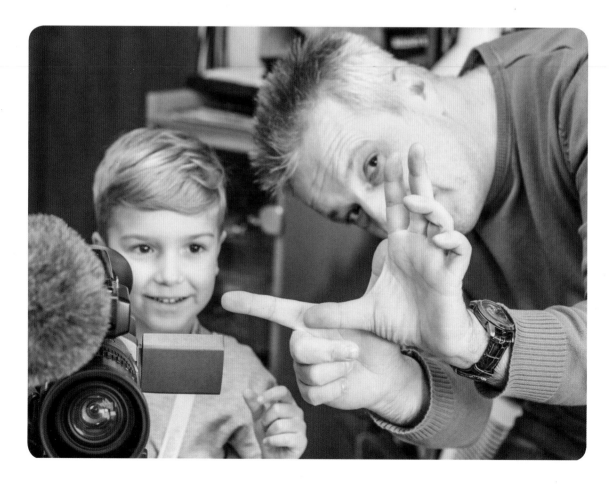

It's easier to remember visual information because our brain can usually associate it with other things stored in our memory. For instance, if we see a picture of a cake, the image may immediately conjure up thoughts of sugar, flour, spoons, or a baker. The fact that the visual image is linked to those other associations makes it easier for our brains to recall memories.

But to make information even more memorable, nothing beats video. Video combines already easy to remember visual images with audio; this union makes video an extremely engaging medium for your brain. In fact, studies show that we tend to remember more than 90 percent of a message if we see it in video form, compared to remembering only 10 percent of it if we read it.

So, use video to your advantage. Make videos of the things you want to remember most, be it kids, pets, or an amazing vacation. Watching a memorable video will not only bring back memories of that moment, but other memories associated with it, as well.

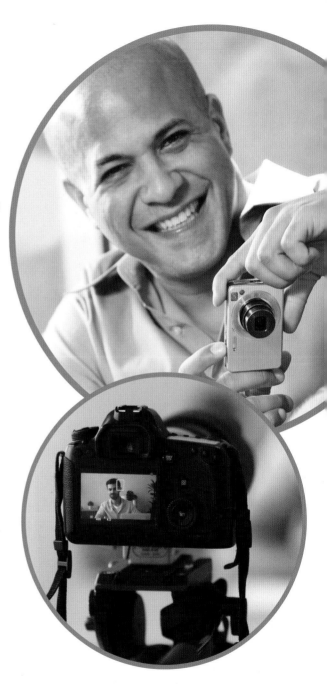

63

Laugh!

We've all heard the old saying, "laughter is the best medicine," but is it really true? Well, surprisingly, this simple action lowers blood pressure, decreases stress, and increases dopamine levels in the brain. And, in the case of your brain, increases in dopamine helps improve memory and recall.

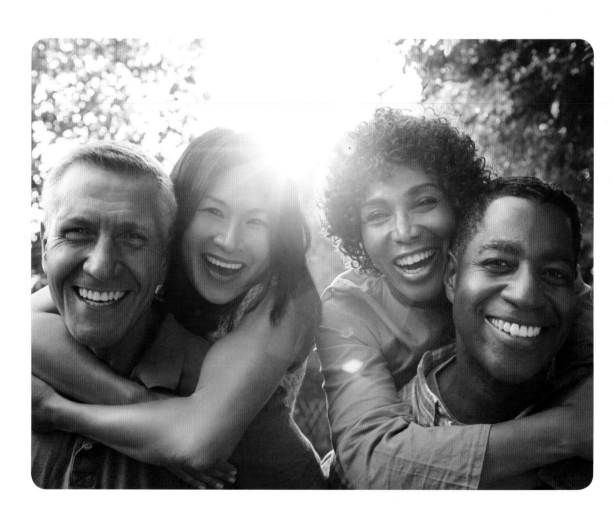

A recent study performed at Loma Linda University in Loma Linda, California, asked two groups of older adults to complete a memory test. One group watched a funny video before the test, and the other did not view the video. Researchers discovered that the group that watched the video had lower levels of stress hormones following the video; the group also had better memory recall, learning ability, and sight recognition than the group that did not watch the video.

Stress hormones, such as cortisol, can decrease the efficiency of the neurons in the hippocampus. By lowering these hormones, laughter can strengthen working memory. An excess of cortisol has also been linked to heart disease, weight gain, and depression; it's no wonder that laughter is considered medicine!

When we're children, laughter tends to come more easily; but as adults, we often take life too seriously. So find reasons to laugh. Watch a funny movie or television show, go to a comedy club, play silly games with your grandchildren, or host a game night for friends. Before you know it, you'll be reaping the benefits of this amazing "medicine."

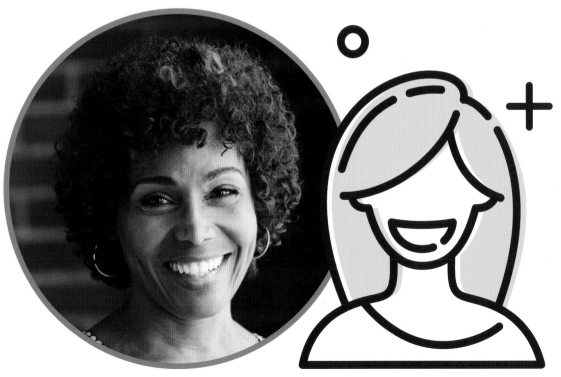

64 Nix Unnecessary Medications

Modern medicine is an amazing thing. Turn on the television or flip through a magazine and you'll see advertisements for drugs and medications that have changed millions of lives for the better, promising relief for everything from depression to psoriasis to cancer. And while it's certainly a privilege to have access to so many options, is it possible we're exposing ourselves to too much of a good thing?

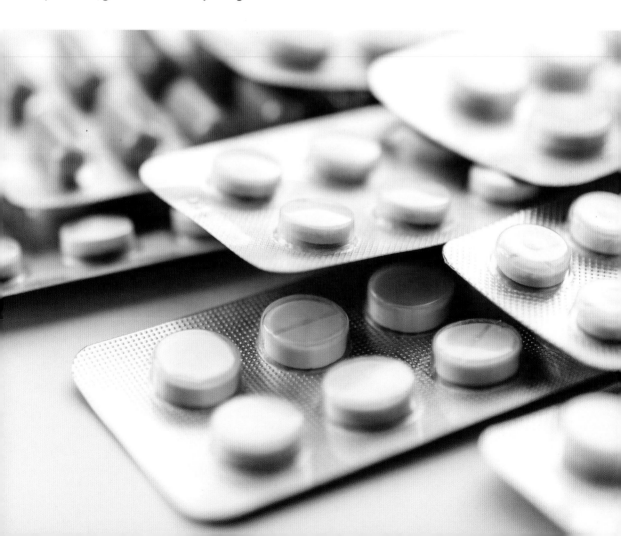

Unfortunately, the answer could be yes. After all, most medications come with side effects, which can range from mildly irritating to unbearable. And if your goal is to keep your brain healthy and sharp for as long as possible, it may be worth it to cut out some of the drugs that are known to cause memory problems.

Some of the drugs to watch out for include:

- Benzodiazepines, or anti-anxiety drugs, which have been linked to dementia

- Prescription sedatives

- Over-the-counter sleep aids, including sedating antihistamines

- Antipsychotics and mood stabilizers

Other drugs that may affect memory include cholesterol-lowering drugs, antidepressants, narcotic painkillers, drugs for hypertension, and antiseizure drugs. Many of these medications have been found to impair memory by blocking pathways in the brain and dampening brain function, especially if used for long periods of time.

Obviously, it is not always feasible to stop taking a medication. Sometimes medication controls symptoms that are harder to bear than any side effects. But if you're worried about the effects a certain medication may be having on your memory, ask your doctor about alternatives.

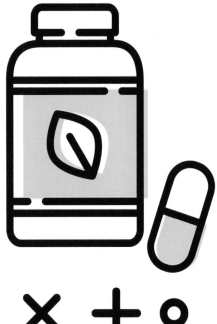

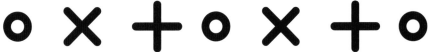

65 Scrutinize Supplements

Given the fact that many medications deplete your body of vital vitamins and minerals, supplements are probably necessary to correct the effects of every-day drug use. There's little question that most people can take a multivitamin without any hazard to their health. But, for everyone, that's not always the case. Like medications, supplements should be scrutinized.

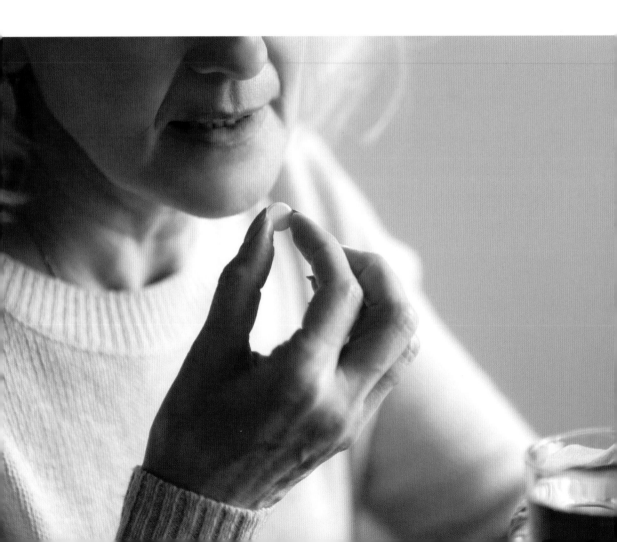

Consider herbal supplements, which are regulated as dietary supplements in this country. That means they do not have to prove their efficacy or safety, according to the Food and Drug Administration. By contrast, prescription and over-the-counter medications must go through a rigorous approval process. That lax attitude toward herbals provides a false sense of security, as consumers may see herbal medicines as harmless and not at all druglike. But nothing could be farther from the truth, especially since people purchase herbals in place of prescription and over-the-counter drugs. That can be a good thing, when properly researched. Just because a pill or potion is derived from a plant doesn't mean it's free of side effects, nor does it make it automatically safe to consume with prescription and over-the-counter medications. And don't forget that the vitamins and minerals you take can potentially have detrimental effects on your body (and memory) when all are taken together. Always consult your doctor about all of the pills, herbs, and vitamin and mineral supplements you take so that he or she has a complete picture.

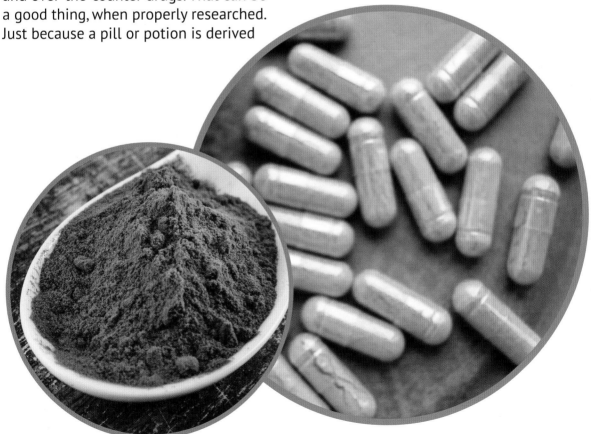

66 Know These Herbs

Plants have been used as nature's primary medicine for thousands of years. People from every continent have used leaves, stems, seeds, fruits, bark, and roots to enhance healing and even memory. Indeed, most modern pharmaceuticals are of plant origin.

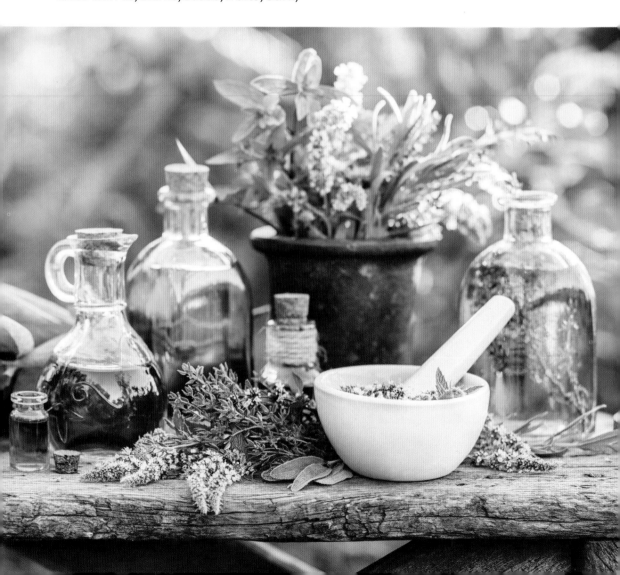

As previously mentioned, some herbs do have side effects when consumed alongside prescription drugs (and even when taken without prescription drugs). Some effects can even be dangerous, especially when taken in high doses. So, if you are taking any prescription medication, don't take any herbs until you've cleared it with your doctor.

Numerous herbs are routinely suggested for treating insomnia (more on sleep later). Most of these herbs appear to have a mild sedating effect that can help reduce stress and anxiety. The herbs most commonly used to promote better sleep, for example, are valerian, hops, passionflower, chamomile, St. John's wort, and lemon balm.

If you decide to experiment with herbs, make sure to follow these basic guidelines:

- Follow recommended doses. More does not mean better.

- Stop using a remedy if you experience any side effects.

- Do not collect herbs from the wild.

- Only buy over-the-counter remedies if the packet states what it contains.

- Follow the directions on the package. Most herbal sedatives should be taken 30 to 45 minutes before bedtime.

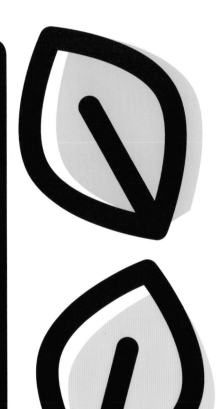

67 Get Enough Vitamin B6

Vitamin B6 is essential to new cell growth. It boosts the immune system while keeping blood glucose levels in check. It also, according to studies, may help improve age-related declines in memory.

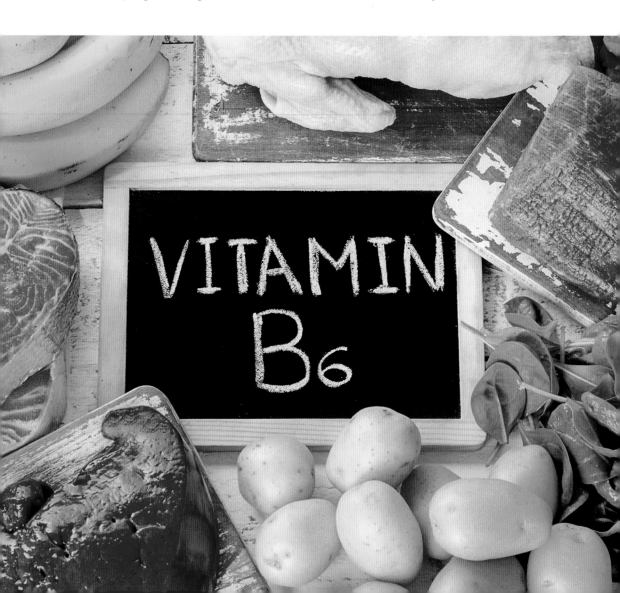

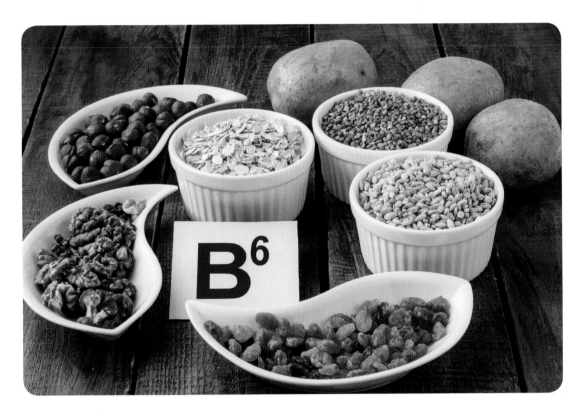

The older you get, the greater the risk of vitamin B6 deficiencies, according to government consumption studies. There are two reasons for this. Since vitamin B6 and protein occur together naturally in foods, people who don't consume enough protein—which is most common among older adults—will also be deficient in vitamin B6. Also, some research suggests that vitamin B6 requirements increase with age because of an increased metabolism of the compound.

Skin problems, anemia, depression, confusion, and even convulsions can occur without adequate vitamin B6. And, since vitamin B6 helps regulate blood sugar, a deficiency in it may boost blood glucose levels as well as levels of insulin.

While the recommended daily intake for adults up to age 50 is 1.3 milligrams (mg) for both men and women, the amount for people over 50 increases to 1.7 milligrams (mg) for men and 1.5 milligrams (mg) for women. Poultry and fish are rich in vitamin B6, along with potatoes and non-citrus fruit.

68 Get Enough Vitamin B12

Vitamin B12 is essential for normal neurologic function and red blood cell formation as well as for fat metabolism. So important is B12 to mental functioning that even borderline deficiencies in it can cause memory loss and other symptoms that mimic dementia. Deficiencies can also cause difficulties with balance, muscle coordination, and manual dexterity. Vitamin B12 deficiencies can cause serious damage to the nervous system, which is irreversible if the condition persists for long.

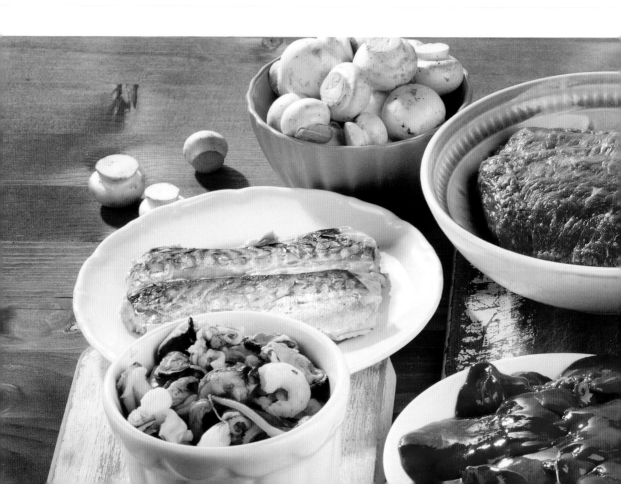

Heading off heart disease, stroke, and peripheral vascular disease—a condition that curtails circulation in your extremities—is another important vitamin B12 function. The vitamin works with two other B vitamins, folate and vitamin B6, to lower homocysteine concentrations in the bloodstream, thus helping prevent these life-threatening diseases.

Although your need for vitamin B12 doesn't increase with age (it remains at 2.4 micrograms daily), your ability to absorb enough of this important vitamin may be compromised. That's because as many as 30 percent of people age 50 and older (and 40 percent of those age 80 and older) have atrophic gastritis, a condition in which the body does not produce enough stomach acid to allow absorption of vitamin B12 from foods. Most people never realize they have this condition.

Aside from fortified foods, beef liver and clams are two of the most concentrated sources of vitamin B12. But fish, meat, poultry, eggs, and many dairy products are also good sources.

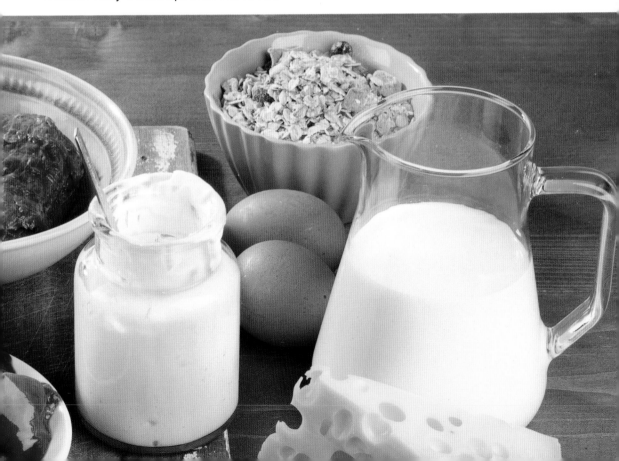

69 Consume Plenty of Folate and Folic Acid

Folate is the naturally occurring variety of a B vitamin found in foods such as legumes, spinach, and orange juice. Folic acid, its synthetic sibling, is added to vitamin pills and to products made from enriched flour, such as bread. Researchers strongly suspect that this B vitamin is linked to mental health, particularly in seniors. Folate even may help prevent depression and preserve mental acumen.

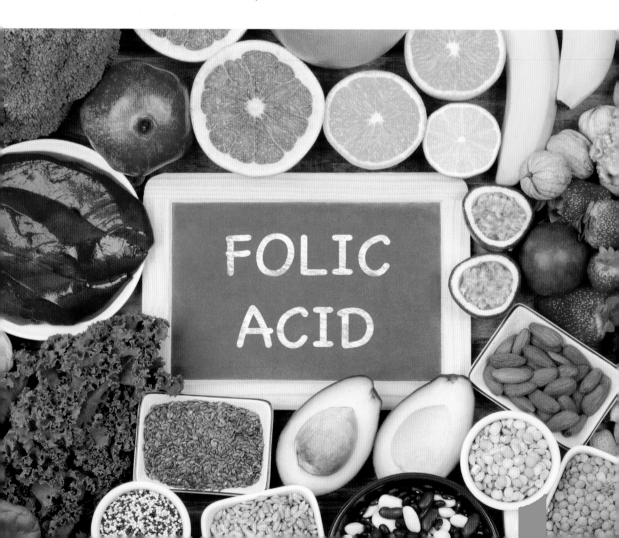

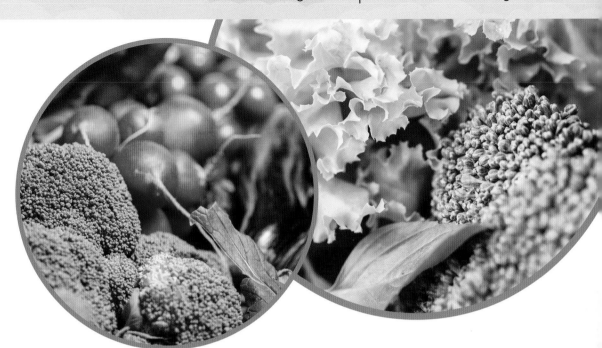

Getting enough folate becomes increasingly important as you age because of its role in the prevention of heart attack, stroke, and circulation problems. Along with vitamins B6 and B12, folate helps rid your bloodstream of excess homocysteine, an amino acid that fosters clogged arteries, blocking the flow of blood to your brain, heart, and extremities.

Without adequate folate, protein production falters, affecting the growth and repair of tissues, which you want to keep in top form as the years go by. While the effects are most noticeable during periods of rapid growth, including infancy and adolescence, a folate shortfall shouldn't be ignored, no matter what your age. As you get older, your cells need all the help they can get to maintain themselves and to replicate in a healthy manner.

Try to meet your daily requirement with a combination of vitamin supplements, fortified foods, and a folate-rich diet. In the case of folate, man-made sources are often better than natural sources because your body absorbs the synthetic form of the vitamin almost twice as efficiently. Folate-rich foods are important to your health, however, and you should still try to eat plenty of plant-based foods. Green vegetables are especially important in order to get enough folate. Nuts, peas, and beans also provide folate.

70 Seek Out Choline

You may not have heard of choline, but this B-like vitamin has been officially recognized as an essential nutrient by the Food and Nutrition Board (FNB) of the National Academy of Science's Institute of Medicine.

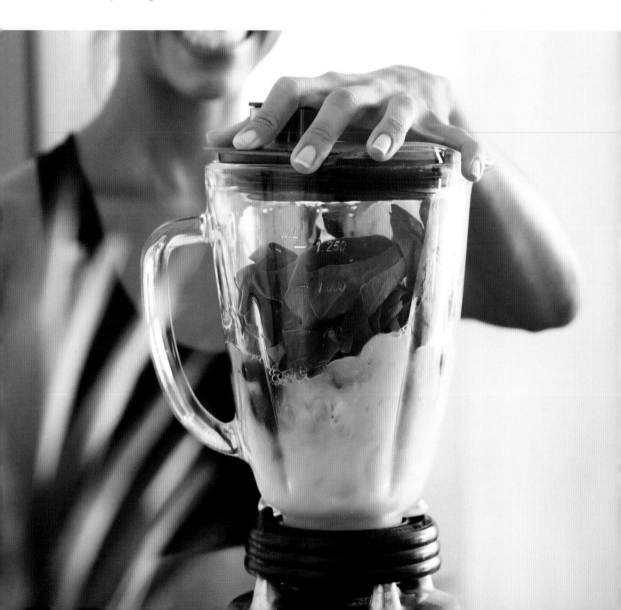

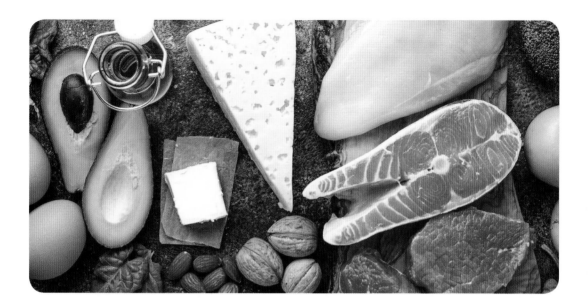

What is choline good for? Well, it serves as the raw material for several substances in the body, including the neurotransmitter acetylcholine, a chemical messenger that ferries information between brain cells and is involved in muscle control. Animal studies show that consuming adequate choline early in life leads to a reduction in the seriousness of memory deficits, such as dementia, when you are older.

Choline is the raw material of cell membranes—the wrappers around cells that preserve their integrity and strength. It is also vital to liver health and may help your body clear excessive levels of homocysteine.

The Food and Nutrition Board sets requirements at 550 milligrams (mg) of choline every day for men age 51 and older and 425 mg for women in that age group. Experts have hinted at an increasing need for choline among older adults but have not set a higher recommended intake for them.

Experts say that milk, eggs, beef, and peanuts head up the list of the richest choline sources. Your best bet for meeting your daily requirement of choline is to eat a wide array of foods, since choline is found to some extent in many different types of foods, including potatoes, whole grains, cauliflower, Brussels sprouts, and broccoli.

71 Take Time for Tea

In ancient China, green tea was thought to provide mental clarity, and now evidence of that is turning up in laboratory studies. Experiments on mice and rat brain cells show that green tea antioxidants seem to prevent the formation of an Alzheimer's-related protein, beta-amyloid, which accumulates in the brain as plaque and leads to memory loss. This finding has been duplicated in a number of other cell-culture experiments. In one of these types of studies the antioxidants in black tea also were protective, although not as much as those found in green tea.

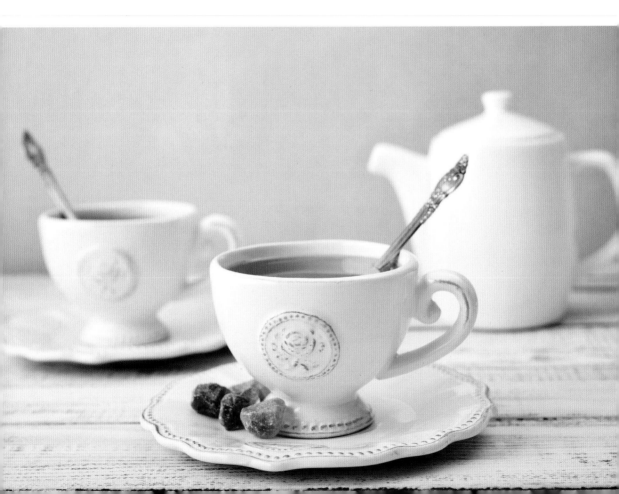

In humans, green tea has been associated with a lower risk of dementia and memory loss. A Japanese study published in the American Journal of Clinical Nutrition surveyed more than 1,000 people older than age 70. Those who drank two or more cups a day of green tea were half as likely to develop dementia and memory loss as those who drank fewer than two cups per week. This effect was much weaker for black and oolong teas.

If you are anemic or have an iron deficiency, drinking tea within an hour or two of eating foods containing iron may make these conditions worse. The pigments in tea and coffee, called tannins, bind to the iron and interfere with its absorption. Green tea also contains vitamin K, which affects blood clotting.

Research into the possible health effects of tea is ongoing and will continue to interest researchers in the years to come. Hidden within tea's leaves there may be clues that could lead to new treatments or even cures for diseases in the future. In the meantime, enjoy tea for the simple joy of its taste and aroma and know that you are protecting your health, too.

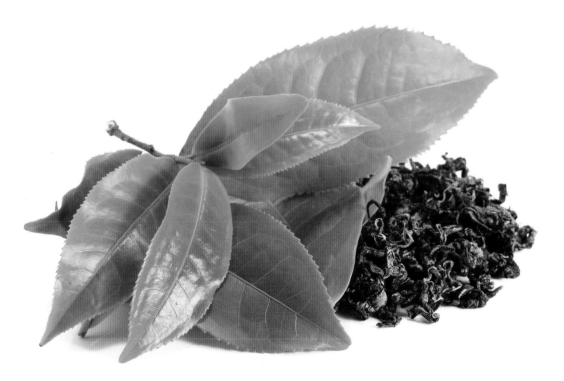

72 Cut Down On Sugar

We all love the occasional (or even regular) sweet, be it a cookie, ice cream cone, piece of cake, or our favorite candy. Sugar, after all, has been around for hundreds of years.

It's a staple of our favorite foods and dishes, and many of us are addicted to sugar in one way or another. It even brings families and friends together.

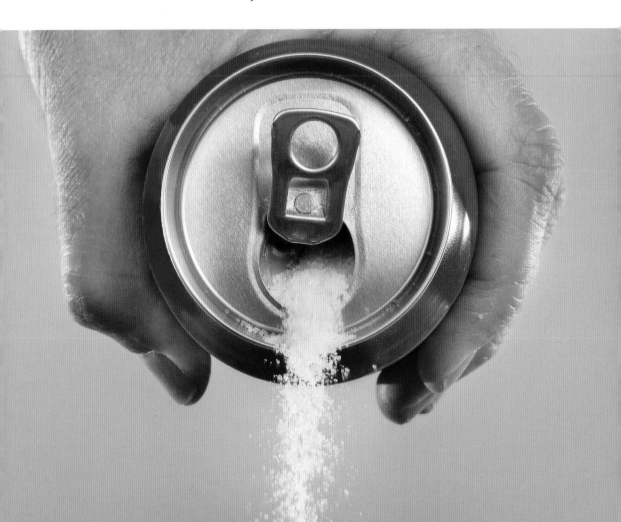

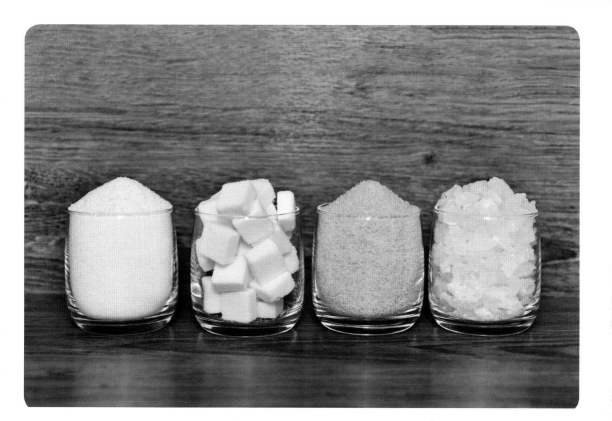

Unfortunately, if you want to keep your brain sharp and memory strong, you'll want to seriously consider cutting down on sugar.

Numerous recent studies have demonstrated that an abundance of sugar can lead to cognitive harm. A study from the Boston University School of Medicine followed more than 4,000 people and found that those who regularly consumed sweetened drinks had worse memory and short-term memory than those who did not. Artificially sweetened beverages may not be much better; consuming even just one sweetened beverage a day can increase the risk of developing a stroke and Alzheimer's disease, according to another study.

What can you consume in place of sugar? Raw honey and dates are excellent substitutes; both are packed with healthy vitamins, including vitamin B6, iron, magnesium, and potassium. The two substitutes are high in calories, however, so keep an eye on your intake.

73 Drink Plenty of Fluids

You need fluids, but your body can't make it in the amounts necessary to sustain life. That makes water absolutely essential, even though it's often shortchanged as a nutrient. You could go for days, even weeks, without food. That long without fluid would spell certain disaster!

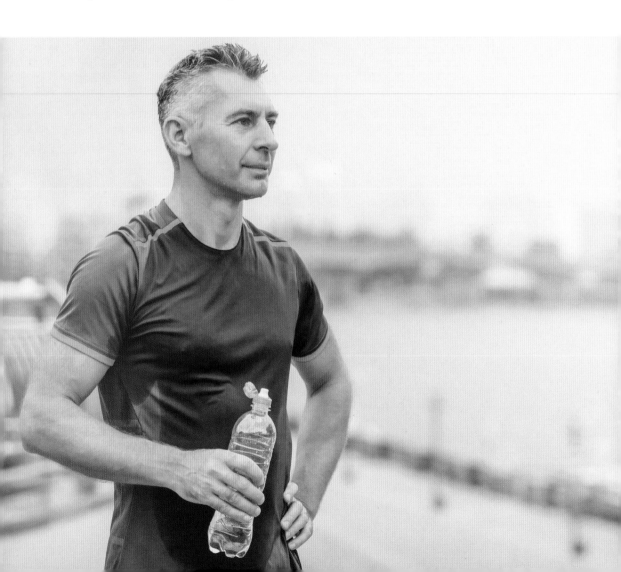

If you're like most people, you take your body for granted, expecting it to always work right. But if you don't feed it enough fluid, all bets are off. Health experts say that older people are prone to nutritional shortcomings that harm their health, and getting too little fluid is one of them. Hot weather and living at high altitudes both push fluid needs even higher.

Moreover, age blunts your ability to detect thirst. For that reason, older people must make a concerted effort to drink more fluids, even when not thirsty, to dodge dehydration. Age also diminishes your body's ability to retain water, making you vulnerable to dehydration. Even mild dehydration can cause confusion, fatigue, headaches, weakness, flushed skin, and light-headedness, symptoms that may be so commonplace that you don't realize fluid loss is the cause.

True, water is absorbed faster than any other fluid and put to use quicker in the body. But you may find drinking water a bit boring. Don't despair. Water isn't the only way to satisfy fluid needs. The recommendation for fluids includes water, seltzer, club soda, milk, juice, and herbal teas.

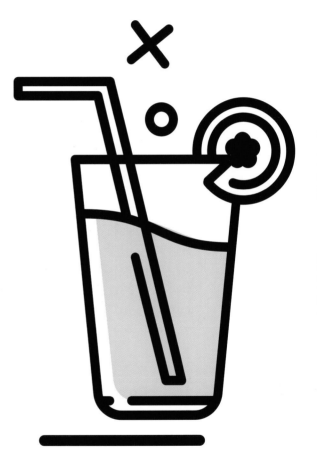

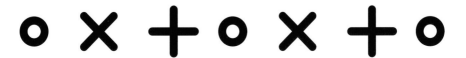

74 Consume Caffeine

Caffeine is a stimulant that increases heart rate, makes you alert, and revs up metabolism. It can also, according to a study published in the journal *Nature Neuroscience,* enhance some memories for more than 24 hours after it is consumed!

Any average coffee drinker knows that the beverage is packed with caffeine; the typical cup (8 ounces) has 110 to 140 milligrams. Most teas natural-ly contain caffeine, but the amount varies depending on the grade and type of tea, whether it is brewed from loose leaves or a tea bag, and how long it is brewed. Black tea has the most caffeine (42 to 72 mg per eight ounces) while green, white, and oolong teas have less (9 to 50 mg per 8 ounces). Decaffeinated teas only have 1 to 4 mg per 8 ounces. Sodas, chocolates, energy drinks, and even medications can also contain caffeine.

If possible, aim to receive caffeine from coffee and tea. They're the healthiest sources of the stimulant!

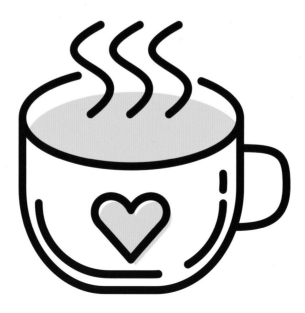

75 Watch Alcohol Intake

Sure, a drink—or two—of alcohol each day is OK, but having more than few beverages can interfere with your brain function (and memory).

Alcohol abuse destroys brain tissue and interferes with the process of absorbing information so that it never enters long-term memory. Indeed, short-term memory loss is often the first sign that alcohol-related neuro-logical damage has occurred; it's also a hallmark of alcoholism. This type of memory loss means a person has difficulty remembering new informa-tion, so the learning process takes longer. Alcohol abuse also reduces higher-level thinking, or the ability to think in abstract terms, which is important for sound decision mak-ing, planning, and other abilities. If untreated, chronic alcohol abusers may even develop a form of dementia marked by disorientation, confused thinking, and severe amnesia.

To put it plainly, excessive drinking actually changes the underlying brain chemistry that controls our abilities and skills. It can, and often does, threaten jobs and relationships. And it can certainly age your brain before its time. If you are struggling with alcohol, help is available. Contact your doctor or hospital for information about local programs and resources.

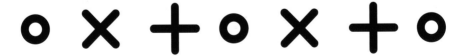

76 Stop Smoking

If you're a smoker, puffing on that cigarette may make you feel reenergized—for a moment. But smoking can actually lower the amount of oxygen that reaches your brain, thereby affecting its functions, including memory and cognition.

In fact, studies have found that smokers score lower on memory tests than do nonsmokers, and smokers who average more than a pack a day have an especially difficult time recalling names and faces. Some studies suggest that smoking can slow your recall ability about as much as having a couple of drinks.

Smoking a pack a day exposes you to a variety of noxious substances, including 1,000 micrograms of toluene, which is highly toxic and can cause confusion and memory loss (as well as other damage). In other words, if you want to prevent premature brain (and body) aging, kick the habit. These days there are all sorts of products and programs that can help.

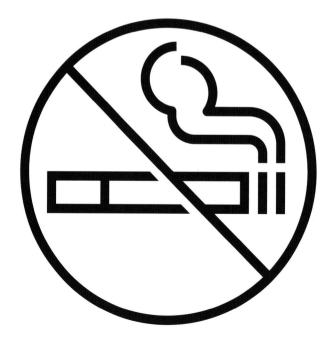

77 Monitor Marijuana Use

When it comes to keeping your brain in tip-top shape no matter your age, there's minimal upside in dabbling in recreational drugs. With marijuana, it's a bit of a double-edged sword.

Marijuana can cause immediate as well as ongoing problems with short-term memory and attention. And both short-term and long-term use of opiates can negatively impact recall, reflexes, attention, concentration, hand-eye coordination, and executive functions. It can even trigger symptoms that are similar to dementia.

However, there has been some research into the effects of the drug on Alzheimer's disease, and the findings are promising. The tetrahydrocannabinol (THC) in marijuana has been shown to inhibit the buildup of proteins in the brains of Alzheimer's patients. When levels of these proteins are abnormally high, as they are in Alzheimer's patients, they can clump together and collect between neurons, disrupting cell function.

Cannabis can also decrease the inflammation that occurs around these amyloid plaques. The other cannabinoids in marijuana show promising effects on the brain, as well. They may help prevent cell death, and may even stimulate cell growth in the area of the brain responsible for memory.

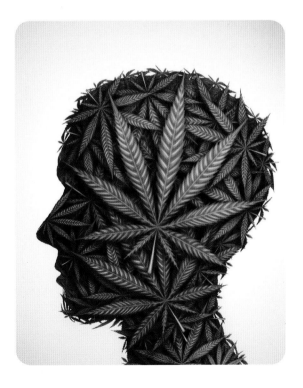

78 Manage Your Weight

Chances are, you weigh more now than you did 10 years ago. But as you get older, it's normal to gain weight, right? It may be normal—if you define "normal" as "common"—but it's not desirable. It's certainly not desirable if you want to keep your memory in good shape, either.

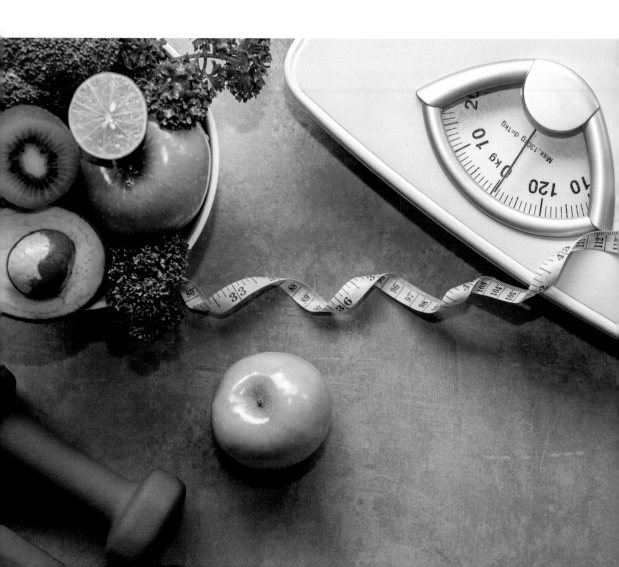

Weight gain is associated with an abundance of adverse health outcomes, from diabetes and heart disease to stroke and cancer. It also, too, can negatively affect your cognition.

A study published in the *British Journal of Nutrition* tracked more than 5,100 adults and found that those with a higher waist-to-hip ratio had poorer memory than their slimmer counterparts. Poorer memory in heavier adults may be due to increased levels of inflammation; high amounts of c-reactive protein (CRP) in the bloodstream, for example, have been associated with decreases in cognitive performance. It's further proof that obesity—or even just being overweight—can be extremely dangerous.

As you're likely well aware, there are a wealth of resources to help you shed excess pounds. Diet, exercise, and the elimination of poor habits are essential.

One thing to remember is that fat is metabolically stagnant. In other words, fat cells require virtually no calories to stay alive. Muscle, on the other hand, is very active metabolically. Muscle cells chew through a lot of calories even when they aren't moving. So when you exercise, and especially when you begin to exercise regularly, your body will burn calories even when you're resting. That makes keeping off excess pounds easier!

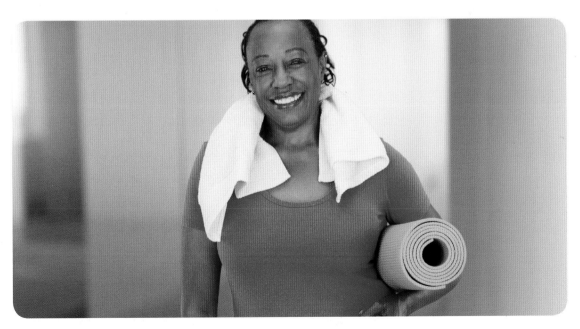

79 Address Your Blood Pressure and Cholesterol Levels

Two evils of the aging body are high blood pressure and high cholesterol. Some people suffer from both; some suffer from just one of the two. Regardless, high blood pressure and high cholesterol levels can wreak havoc on the body—and, subsequently, your memory.

Between 40 and 50 percent of people over the age of 65 have high blood pressure, yet scientists are not sure why. In about 95 percent of the cases the cause remains a mystery. The decreased elasticity of the blood vessels as we age may be at least partially responsible for high blood pressure, but lifestyle may be equally, if not more, responsible.

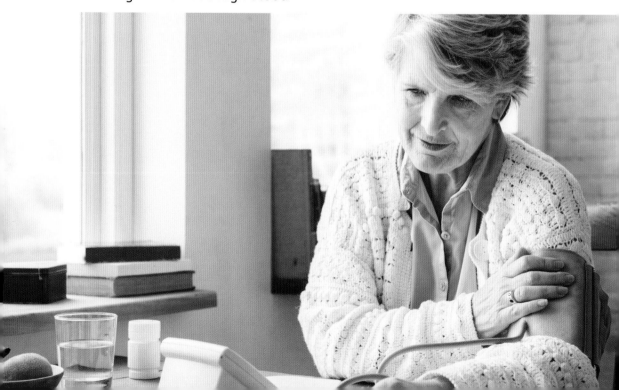

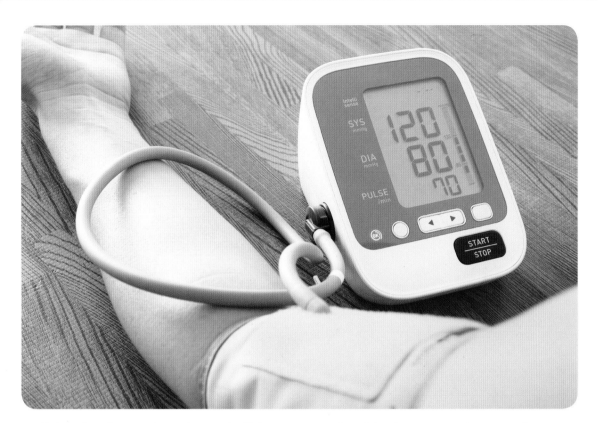

Scientists know that plaque buildup increases with age but is exacerbated by elevated total cholesterol levels and by elevated LDL (low density lipoproteins, the "bad" cholesterol) levels in the blood. A diet rich in saturated fat and cholesterol and low in fiber coupled with a sedentary lifestyle contribute to high blood levels of total cholesterol and LDL cholesterol.

Quite simply, you must control your blood pressure and "bad" cholesterol levels. One study pinpointed mid-life high blood pressure as the major reason for thinning nerve tissue and reduced brain volume of people in their 70s. Researchers found that along with cigarette smoking, excessive alcohol consumption, and mismanaged diabetes, high blood pressure speeds up the normal changes seen in the aging brain.

If you have high blood pressure and/or high cholesterol, make sure to get screened regularly and talk to your doctor about how to control these conditions.

80 Take Care of Your Teeth and Gums

Regular brushing and flossing are simple things you can do to protect your health. Spending just five minutes each day with your teeth and gums can dramatically improve your well-being, not to mention your breath. But maintaining excellent oral hygiene may even be good for keeping your memory intact.

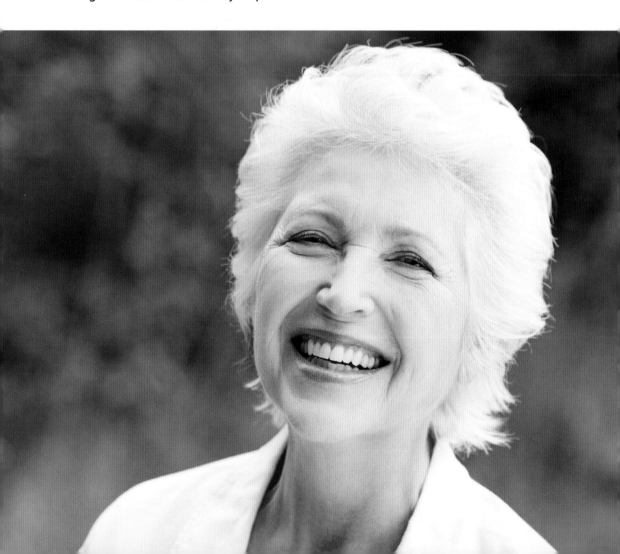

A study by researchers at West Virginia School of Dentistry examined the oral health, memory, and blood work of patients over the age of 60. Researchers found that the men and women who scored the worst on the memory test had poorer oral hygiene and more gum disease-causing bacteria than those who fared better.

Another study by the Chung Shan Medical University in Taiwan found that chronic inflammation, especially periodontitis, could promote the development of Alzheimer's disease. The researchers concluded that people over the age of 70 who had a gum disease for more than 10 years were 70 percent more likely to develop dementia than those with better oral health.

In addition to daily brushing and flossing, calcium and vitamin D play important roles in keeping bones and teeth strong and healthy. Fortified milk, breakfast cereals, and fish are excellent sources of these two nutrients.

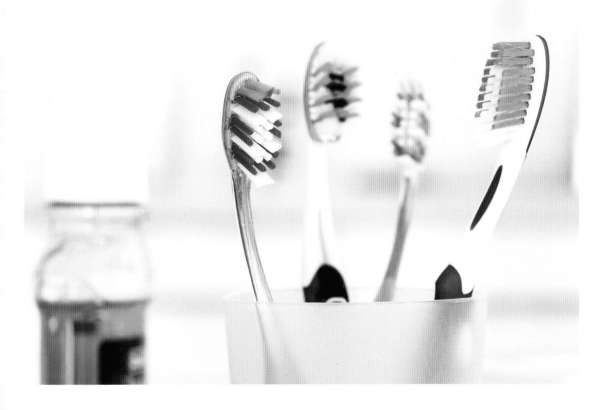

81 Control Chronic Pain

At some point, it's almost a guarantee that you'll suffer (if you haven't already) from chronic pain. In fact, the Centers for Disease Control and Prevention has estimated that about 50 million American adults suffer from this debilitating disorder; the actual number, however, could be quite higher. Chronic pain can affect mood, sleep, and work performance. There's little surprise, then, that it can also affect your memory.

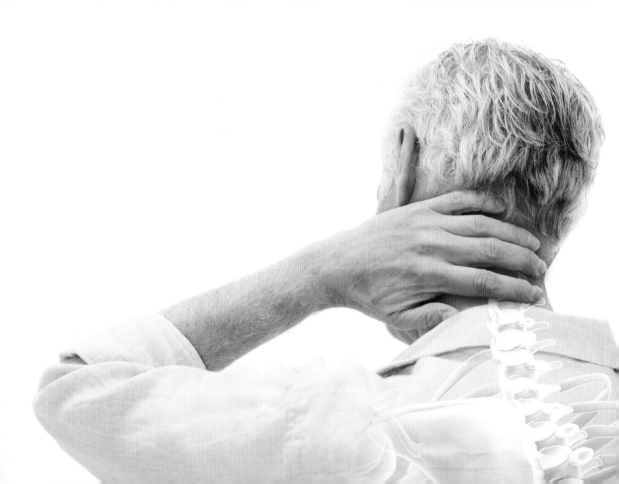

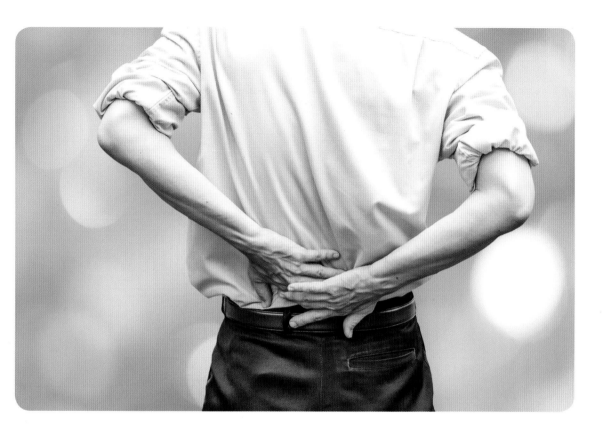

Numerous studies show that the vast majority of people with chronic pain report disruptions in memory and attention. That's because pain can impair the hippocampus, impeding growth and neuron development. One study from the University of Alberta found that a majority of chronic pain patients who did not receive a pain-reliving treatment performed far worse on verbal memory and spatial tests than when they did receive the treatment.

Depending on your type of pain, there are a variety of different treatment options. Exercise and diet are essential, but alternative ideas (including acupuncture, biofeedback, and meditation, all of which are covered in the remaining pages of this book) can be equally attractive options.

82 Check Your Hearing

Do you find yourself saying "what?" more often? Maybe you don't like crowds as much since you can't detect the nuances of conversations that well. Hearing loss is one of the most common complaints of getting older, especially for men, who are more prone to hearing loss at any age.

Aging produces a progressive hearing loss at all frequencies, known as presbycusis. After age 55, your ability to detect changes in the pitch of sounds drops off dramatically, which can make your speech less understandable to others.

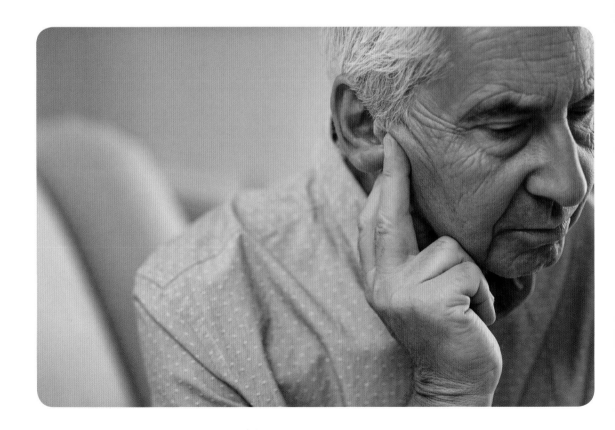

Hearing loss can an isolate you from friends and family and limit your social involvement and enjoyment of life—which, in turn, can have profound effects upon your mental state and memory.

It's certain that the loss of hair cells is what diminishes hearing the most. Hair cells are part of the inner ear that help transmit impulses to a nerve that transfers them to your brain for processing. Nerve damage, injury, exposure to loud noise, and certain medications can cause hair cell loss.

If you strain to hear others in a noisy background, find yourself asking others to repeat themselves, or consistently misunderstand the speech of others, discuss your hearing loss with your doctor.

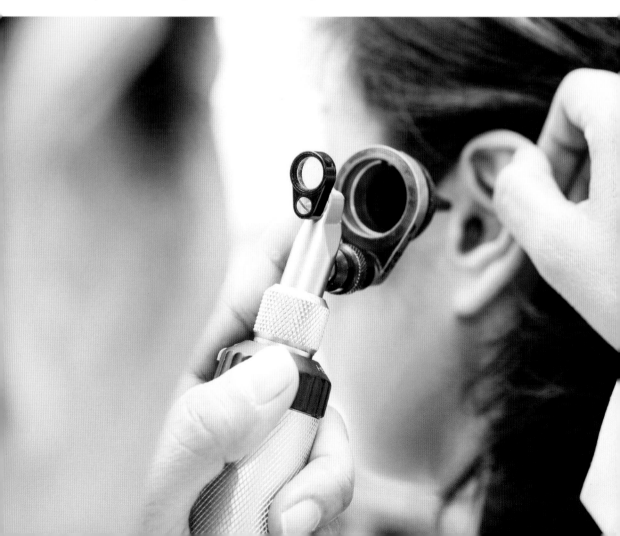

83 Protect Your Head From Injury

Any discussion of the ways in which you can preserve youthful cognitive functioning as the years go by would not be complete without emphasizing the importance of shielding your brain from head injuries. Such assaults can cause lasting physical and cognitive damage!

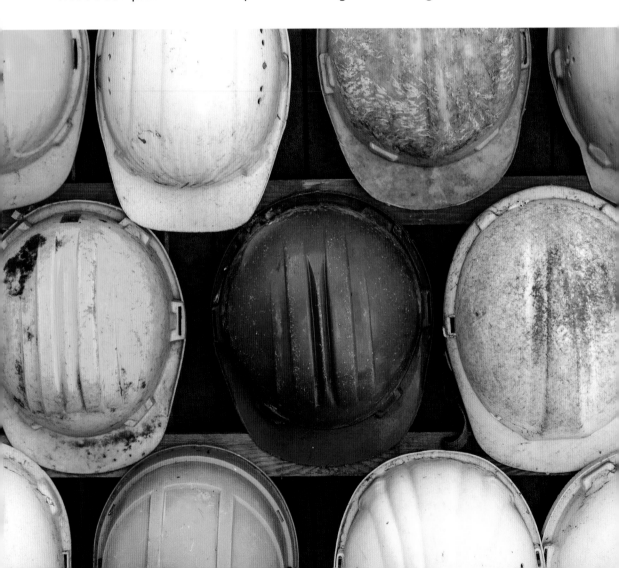

If you want to make sure that your mind stays as sharp as possible for as long as possible, it's essential that you do all you can to avoid injury to your head. A growing body of research links head injury—especially the kind that causes traumatic brain injury (TBI)—to lasting and sometimes devastating problems with cognition, memory, and other brain functions. It is also linked to a higher risk of Alzheimer's disease and other forms of dementia. It makes sense to protect your head.

Awareness of the potential dangers of head injury has been growing in the United States. That increased attention is likely due at least in part to the expanding population of older Americans, who have an increased incidence of falls, as well as to the much-publicized struggles of several retired professional athletes who suffered traumatic brain injury from repeated head blows during their playing days.

Falls are the leading cause of TBIs, and they hit older individuals especially hard. More than 80 percent of TBIs in adults aged 65 and older are the result of falls. Falls also prompt the most hospitalizations for TBI in people 45 years of age and older. Aging can take a toll on eyesight, mobility, balance, and reaction time, increasing the risk of falls.

So the next time that you ride a bike or scooter, make sure to grab that helmet. Your brain will thank you!

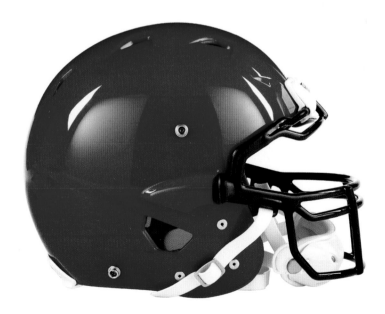

84 Don't Skimp Out On Sleep

Though many years of research have enlightened us to important aspects of sleep and why it's important, there is still much we don't know.

Well, there are some things that we do know:

• Sleep restores our mental energy. As we sleep, we tend to store and reorganize information we have accumulated throughout the day. (The brain doesn't shut down after all!) This regular mental housekeeping during sleep appears to enhance learning and creativity.

• Sleep is an important time when the body heals muscle tissue and restores itself. Our metabolic activity is at its lowest during deep sleep, providing an opportunity for the body to rebuild and heal. This is crucial both during the growth years of childhood and during adult life.

• During sleep, our brain waves slow down considerably compared to our waking state. This slowing of brain waves creates a combination of light and deep sleep that cycles repeatedly through the night. Our degree of refreshment the next day depends on how these cycles play out while we sleep.

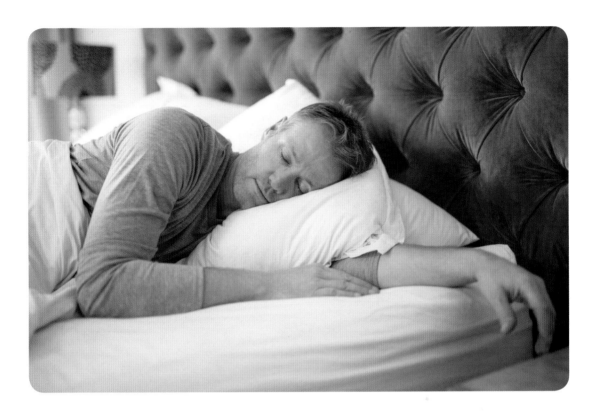

Sounds important, right? That's because it is, and sleep is essential for improving our memory.

Although sleep needs vary somewhat among individuals, there is a certain minimum amount of sleep humans require. Research indicates that to perform adequately at home and on the job—in other words, without falling asleep at the wheel, making dumb mistakes due to tiredness, or being cranky and impatient with others— and also to avoid the in-creased health risks of chronic sleep deficiency, most adults need seven to eight hours of sleep each night. Some adults called "short sleepers" naturally require less than six hours of sleep at night. At the other end of the spectrum are "long sleepers" who need nine or more hours of sleep per night.

Luckily, there are a plethora of strategies available to prepare your body for restful sleep. Read on to learn more!

85 Establish a Bedtime Ritual

Most of us begin our day with a morning routine. It helps us prepare ourselves physically and mentally for the day. So why not establish a bedtime routine that helps to prepare you for sleep? The purpose of a bedtime ritual is to send a signal to your body and mind that it's time to sleep.

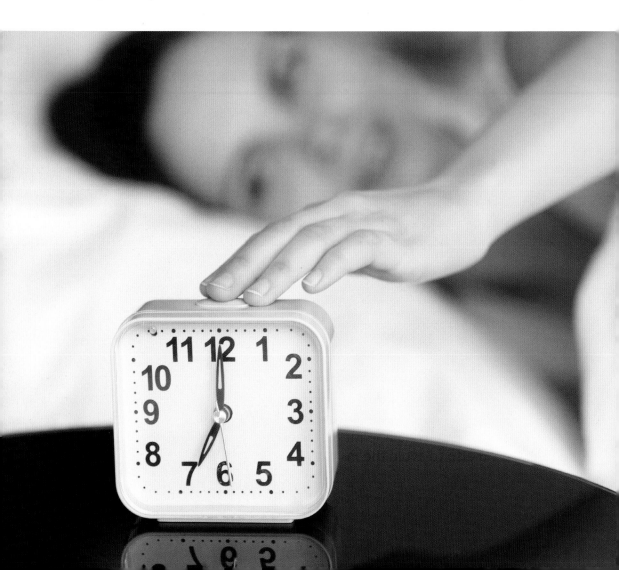

You probably already have some regular bedtime habits, even if you haven't realized it. Brushing and flossing your teeth, lowering the thermostat, and setting your alarm clock may all be part of your evening routine. To help you get to sleep, you should perform these activities in the same manner and order every night.

Avoid activities that are stimulating or laden with emotion right before bedtime. Begin those types of activities earlier in the evening, and end them in time to go unhurriedly through your bedtime routine. Establishing some type of bedtime ritual also provides closure to your day and allows you to go to bed and sleep with a quieter body and mind.

Make a standing appointment with your pillow. It's often too easy to put off bedtime to do one more chore, watch one more episode, or read one more page. So try writing or typing "bedtime" into the same time slot of your planner or calendar every day. It might seem a bit silly at first, but seeing your bedtime written down—just like your other appointments—may help reinforce its importance. Having a set end-time to your day clearly noted in your calendar may also help you avoid overscheduling or planning activities too late in the evening.

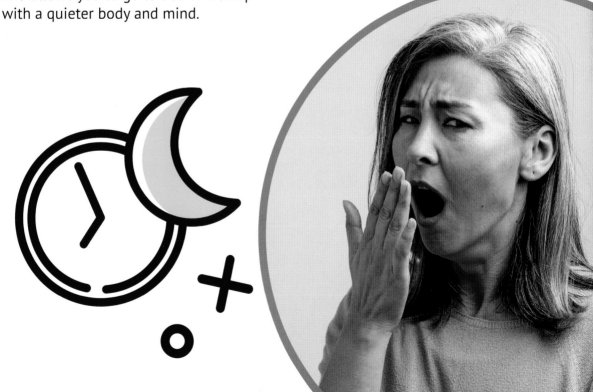

86 Eat and Drink Wisely

How much of a direct effect diet has on sleep is unclear. It's safe to say, though, that a balanced, varied diet full of fresh fruits, vegetables, whole grains, and low-fat protein sources can help your body function optimally and help ward off chronic conditions. And since chronic diseases and the drugs required to treat them can interfere with sleep, eating wisely can help your sleep (and memory).

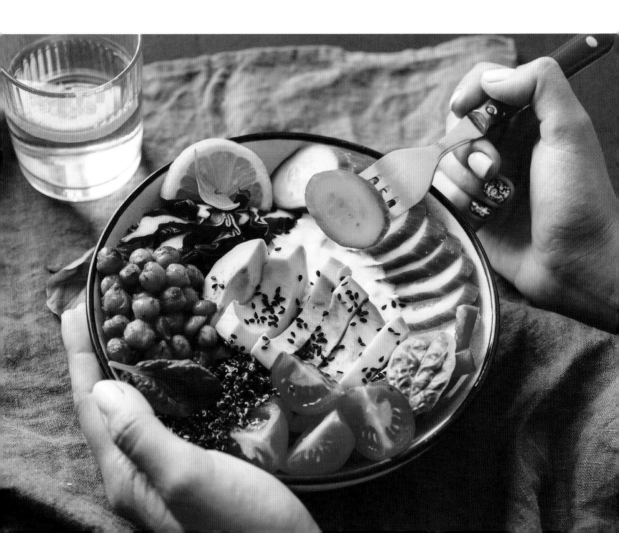

Adjusting your eating routine may also help you get a better night's sleep. Most Americans eat a light breakfast, a moderate lunch, and a large meal in the evening. Yet leaving the largest meal to the end of the day may not be the best choice, since it can result in uncomfortable distension and possibly heartburn when you retire for the night. You might want to try reversing that pattern for a more sleep-friendly meal plan:

- Eat a substantial breakfast. Because you are breaking your nighttime fast and consuming the nutrients you will need for energy throughout the morning, breakfast should be your largest meal of the day. Whole-grain breads and cereals, yogurt, and fruit are just a few examples of good breakfast choices.

- Opt for a moderate lunch. Choose brown rice, pasta, or whole-grain bread and a serving of protein—fish, eggs, chicken, meat, or beans.

- Finish with a light dinner. It is particularly important to eat lightly for your evening meal in order to prepare for a good night's sleep. Plan to finish your meal at least two hours before going to bed, preferably longer.

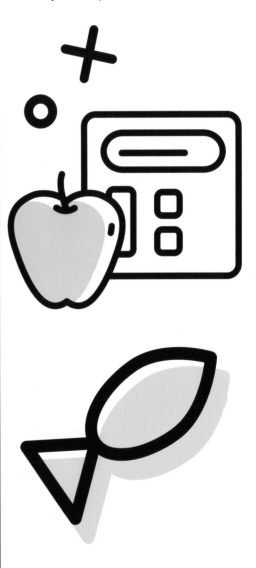

87 Check for Sleep Apnea

At least 25 million Americans suffer from sleep apnea, a potentially life-threatening disorder that causes a person to stop breathing during sleep. Sleep apnea can strike people of any age, but it is most frequently seen in men over 40, especially those who are overweight or obese. The word apnea means "without breath."

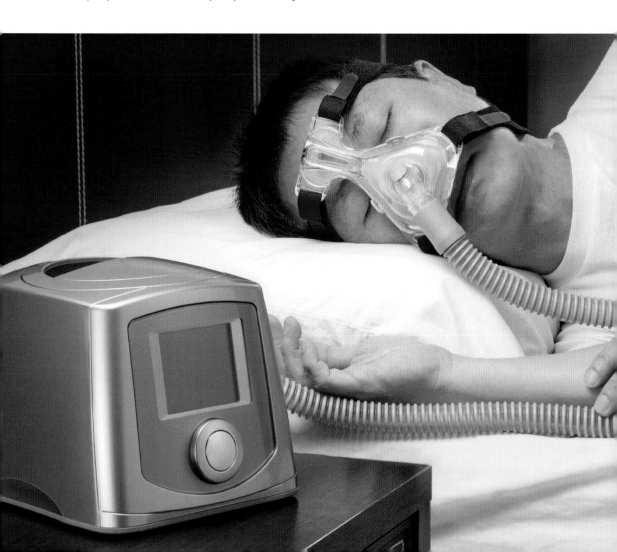

Because people who have sleep apnea frequently go from deeper sleep to lighter sleep during the night, they rarely spend enough time in deep, restorative stages of sleep. Not only do people with sleep apnea struggle with constant fatigue, but they are also at greater risk for accidents, high blood pressure, heart attacks, and other health conditions.

There are several types of sleep apneas. Obstructive sleep apnea (OSA) occurs when the airway collapses or becomes blocked during sleep. Central sleep apnea (CSA) occurs when the brain fails to send proper signals to the muscles that control breathing. Complex or mixed sleep apnea is a combination of the two conditions. Breathing interruptions result from both airway obstruction and faulty brain signaling.

Doctors diagnose sleep apnea based on medical and family histories, symptoms, a physical exam, and results from a sleep study (polysomnography) and/or other tests. Your doctor will determine if your sleep study should be conducted at a sleep center or at home with a portable diagnostic device.

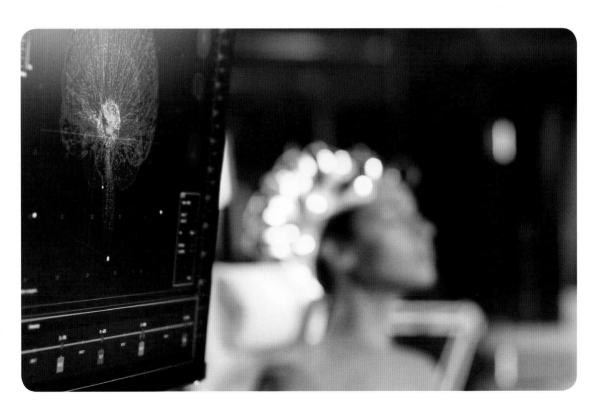

88 Take a Warm Bath

One popular way to relax the body and slow down the mind is a warm bath, and you may find it fits the bill for you. But you may want to do some experimenting with your timing. Some people find a nice hot bath just before bed makes them drowsy and ready to drop into sleep.

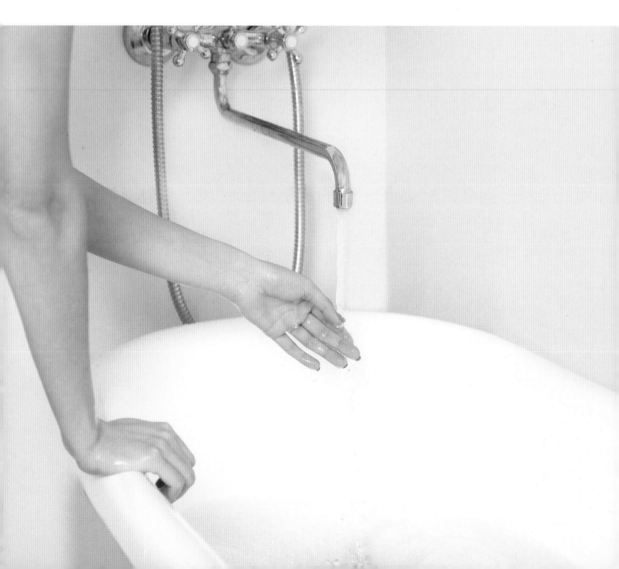

On the other hand, some people find that a hot bath is actually stimulating or that it makes them too uncomfortably warm when they slip into bed. If you find a just-before-bed bath makes it harder for you to fall asleep, consider taking the bath earlier, a couple of hours before bed. An earlier bath may enhance the gradual drop in body temperature that normally occurs at night and help trigger drowsiness.

You can make your own soothing bath with very little effort. Consider making your bath more relaxing by:

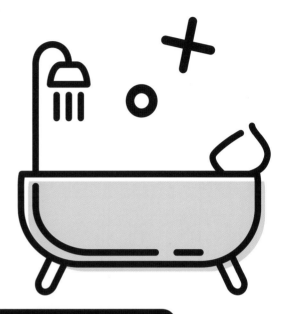

• Dimming the lights and/or using candles to create a calming atmosphere

• Playing soft music in the background

• Reading pleasurable material

• Adding 2 cups of Epsom salts to the bathwater to ease sore or tired muscles

• Laying back and using a towel or waterproof pillow to support your head

89 Make Your Bed a Haven

Most of us think of our bed as a place to sleep. But many people also use their bed for watching television, listening to the radio, talking on the phone, texting, answering e-mails, eating, reading, or playing games. If you really want to sleep better, however, you shouldn't do any of these non-sleep activities in bed. When you do, the bed and bedroom can become associated with these activities rather than with sleep. Instead, you want to condition your mind and body to become drowsy and ready for sleep when you get into your bed, not ready and alert for a chat with a friend or a drama on TV.

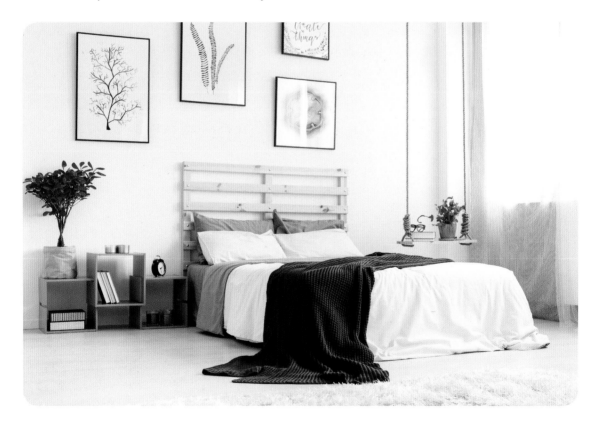

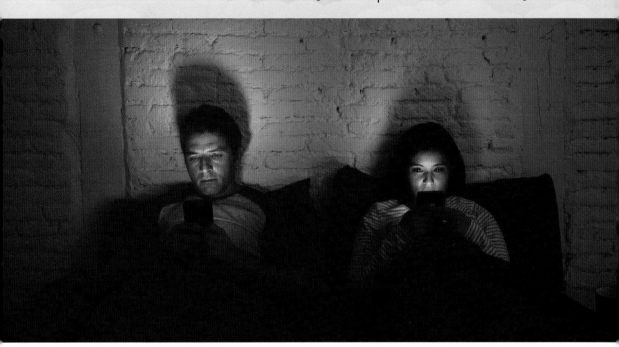

Some people even go so far as to do work in bed. While this practice may help you catch up on paperwork, it can seriously disrupt your sleep. When you do work in bed, all of the associated stress becomes related to the bed and bedroom. Just getting into bed at night may subsequently cause your heart rate to increase, your muscles to tighten, and your thoughts to race. Whether you consciously realize it, the sheets, blankets, and pillows can become associated with your work. Their very sight and smell may cause thoughts of work to flood your mind as you try to fall asleep.

The single exception to the rule about banning non-sleep activities in bed may be sex. We say "may be," because it depends on the effect that sex has on you and your bed partner. For some people, sexual activity is very relaxing and tiring and tends to make them sleepy. If that's the case for both partners, then having sex before sleep may be just the ticket for a restful night.

However, some people find sexual activity actually refreshes and energizes them, making them more alert. And, for some folks, relationship problems, frustrations, or negative feelings about sex can make it far from pleasant or relaxing. For couples in which either partner finds sexual activity too stimulating or too fraught with negative emotions to be conducive to sleep, sex might best be left for another time and even a different room.

90 Nap Sparingly

Some people swear by naps; others find that napping during the day disrupts their sleep at night. The urge to nap is greatest about eight hours after we awaken from a night's sleep. This is when our body temperature begins the first of two daily dips (the other, more dramatic dip, occurs at night). A short nap in the early to middle afternoon can bring a renewed sense of energy and alertness. A nap in the late afternoon or early evening, on the other hand, can disrupt your sleep cycle and make it difficult to fall asleep when you retire for the night.

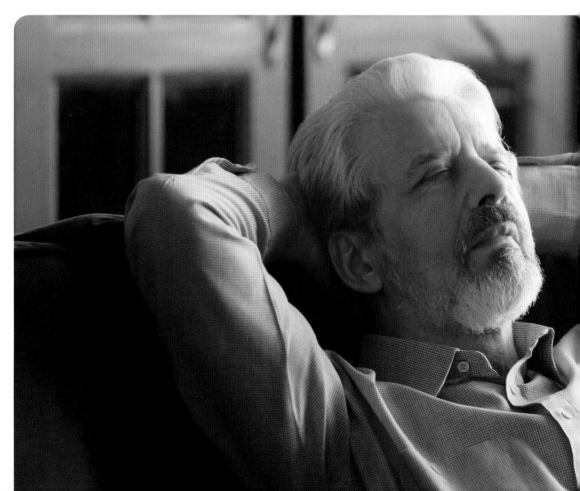

To benefit most from a nap, take it no later than mid-afternoon and keep it under 30 minutes. If you nap for a longer period, your body lapses into a deeper phase of sleep, which can leave you feeling groggy when you awaken. If you are severely sleep-deprived and can't go on without a nap, it is better to sleep for a longer time to allow yourself to go through one complete sleep cycle. An average sleep cycle takes about 90 minutes in most people.

If you find you need a nap every day, take it at the same time so your body can develop a rhythm that incorporates the nap. It's also possible to use naps to temper the negative effects of an anticipated sleep deficit. For instance, if you know you are going to be up late because of special plans, take a prolonged nap of two to three hours earlier in the day. This has been shown to reduce fatigue at the normal bedtime and improve alertness, although it may throw off your normal sleep rhythm temporarily.

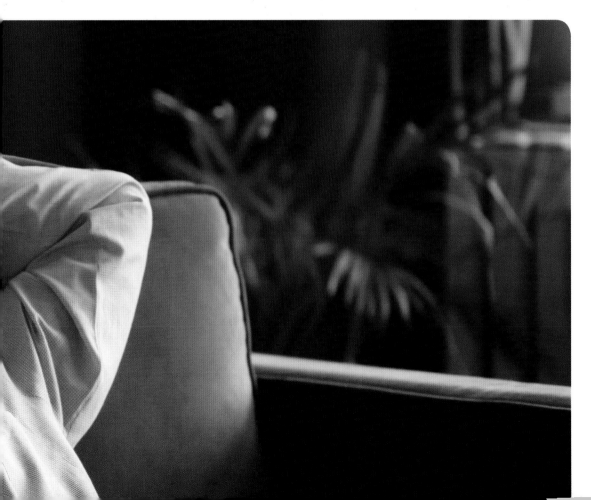

91 Brighten Your Morning

Light tells the brain it is time to wake up. That's probably obvious to anyone who has had to turn on a light in the middle of the night and then has had trouble getting back to sleep. What may not be so obvious is that exposure to light at other times, particularly in the early morning, can actually help you sleep at night.

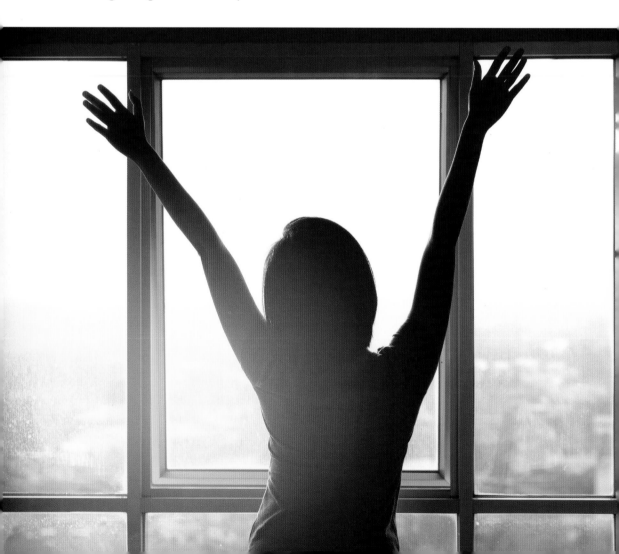

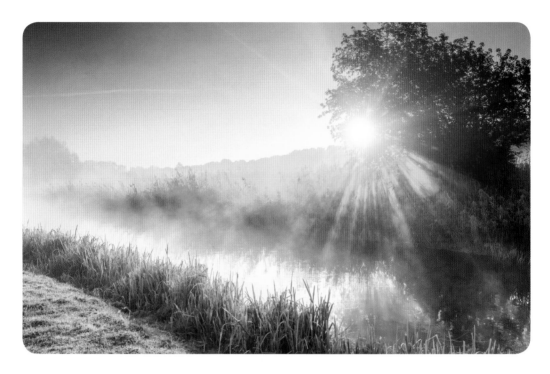

How does morning light improve sleep? The light helps to regulate your biological clock and keep it on track. This internal clock is located in the brain and keeps time not all that much differently from your wristwatch. There does, however, appear to be a kind of forward drift built into the brain. By staying up later and, more importantly, getting up later, you enforce that drift, which means you may find you have trouble getting to sleep and waking up when you need to. To counter this forward drift, you need to reset your clock each day, so that it stays compatible with the earth's 24-hour daily rhythm—and with your daily schedule. Exposing yourself to light in the morning appears to accomplish this reset.

Many factors can affect our biological clock, but light appears to be the most important. The timing of exposure is crucial; the body clock is most responsive to sunlight in the early morning, between 6:00 and 8:30 a.m. Exposure to sunlight later does not provide the same benefit. The type of light also matters, as does the length of exposure. Direct sunlight outdoors for at least 30 minutes produces the most benefit.

92 Manage Stress

It's important to dispel the myth that you can avoid stress. If you breathe, you are going to encounter life situations that bring stress. Since you can't avoid it, the best option is to learn to manage it. One key to managing stress is assessing what you have control over and what you don't.

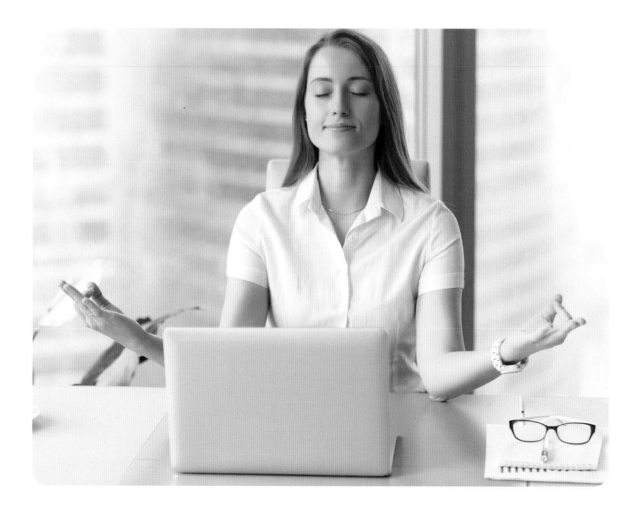

For instance, if your boss has set an unrealistic deadline for a project, you may have little or no control over changing that. But you do have control over how you respond to that deadline. And your response to a given situation is what you want to focus on as you seek to manage stress. You can choose to do certain things and not others. This ability to choose puts you in control.

Professional therapists who specialize in stress reduction will tell you that your body is the best guide to determining when you are feeling stressed. If you pay attention to how you feel physically and emotionally, you can often intervene before stress begins to interfere with sleep.

What does stress management during the day have to do with sleeping well at night? Plenty. Have you ever had the unpleasant experience of crawling into bed exhausted, wanting to put a terrible day behind you, and spending the next few hours tossing and turning as you go over every detail of your day? That is stress at work on your mind. All of those emotions and thoughts throughout the day that were not dealt with at the time can work their way to the surface in the quiet of night.

In addition, the more you dwell on the upsetting events, the greater the effect on your body. When it senses stress, the brain sends a message to the body to release hormones that heighten alertness and prepare it for action. This is known as the fight-or-flight response. By learning to deal with stressors in your life more immediately during the day, you are less likely to be kept awake by them at night.

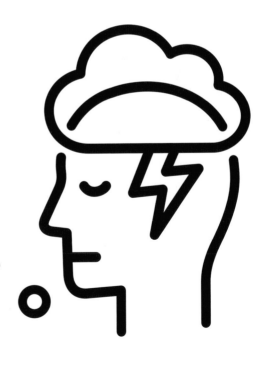

93 Actively Relax

An excellent way to quiet your body and mind before bedtime is to use one of the active relaxation techniques. These techniques help you to deliberately clear your mind of intrusive thoughts, wring the tension from your body, and put yourself into a peaceful state.

One powerful relaxion technique is progressive muscle relaxation (PMR). When you tense a muscle for a few seconds, it naturally wants to relax. That is how PMR works.

You start at your toes and deliberately tense one muscle group at a time, progressively working your way up the body. To prepare, lie on your back on the floor or on a couch or recliner in a room other than your bedroom. Begin by scrunching your toes as hard as you can for 10 seconds, while keeping the rest of your body relaxed. Then relax your toes, and tighten and release your calf muscles, again leaving your other muscles relaxed. Continue through the other muscle groups.

Take your time at it; performing the muscle relaxation one time, from toes to head, should take at least 20 minutes. You should feel very relaxed when you finish. If you don't, repeat the entire cycle one more time.

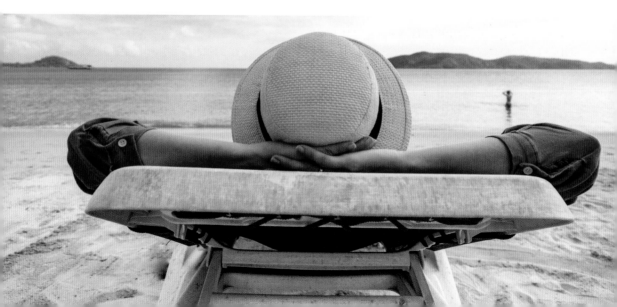

Practice
Abdominal Breathing
94 and Visualization

Another popular relaxation technique is abdominal breathing. Rhythmic breathing is one of the best ways to help your body relax, and there are many variations. This particular technique appears simple, but you'll need a little practice to do it properly.

First, lie down on your back and begin to breathe normally. Now place your hand on your lower abdomen, just at your belt line, and slowly fill your lungs with air to the point that you can feel this portion of your abdomen rise. Take in as much air as you can and hold it for a couple of seconds. Then slowly release all the air in your lungs. Try to pay attention to nothing but the slow intake and release of air, the rhythmic rising and falling of your abdomen. Repeat this eight to 10 times.

Visualization is another powerful relaxation exercise. Imagine your favorite vacation spot. Maybe it's sitting on the sand with your bare feet being massaged by the ocean surf, or scuba diving off some coral reef. Alternately, think of an activity you find especially relaxing: drawing, cooking, hiking, walking your dog, even shopping. The idea behind visualization is to use your imagination to envision something that tells your mind to enjoy itself instead of being focused on some worry or concern.

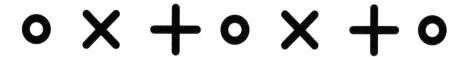

95 Try Meditation

Meditation is an excellent way to balance your physical, emotional, and mental states. Mindfulness meditation can help you pull your mind away from concerns about the past or future and focus on the present moment. Meditation is not so much an emptying of the mind as it is a calming of the mind. One of the first thing things people realize when they begin meditating is how fast and furious their thoughts bombard them when they try to be still.

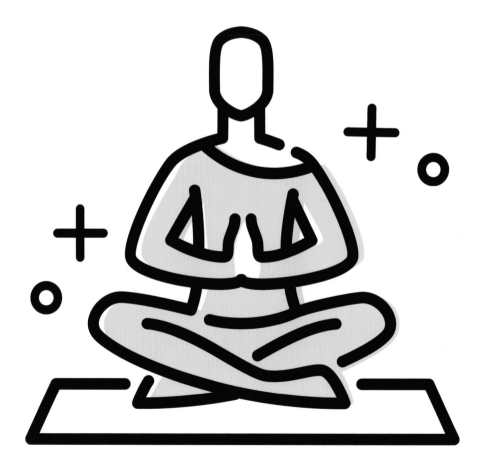

During meditation, the pulse rate slows, blood pressure falls, blood supply to the arms and legs increases, levels of stress hormones drop, and brain waves resemble a state of relaxation found in the early stages of sleep. These are all physical changes that can be brought about by learning to clear your mind of clutter and focus your thoughts. You can use meditation to clear and refresh your mind during the day or help you relax at night in preparation for sleep.

Being mindful means being completely present to the feelings, sensations, and experiences of the moment. It means putting away watches and phones and devices and tuning into nature or the sound of your own breath. It means having no sense of worry, need, fear, demand, or expectation of what should be and instead allowing life to unfold as is. Mindfulness requires no equipment or membership.

Despite a popular myth, you don't need to contort your body into a cross-legged lotus position to meditate. A sitting or lying position will do just fine. (If you choose a sitting position, keep your spine straight but your shoulders relaxed.) It also helps to have a quiet place where you won't be distracted or disturbed. Once you're situated, close your eyes and breathe slowly, feeling the air enter your lungs. Next, exhale slowly, feeling the air leave your body. Keep the focus on your breathing. If your mind wanders off, gently bring your focus back to your breathing. You want your attention to remain on your breathing to keep you in the present moment. This way you won't be distracted by past or future events that may carry your mind away and possibly bring anxiety.

Practice this for 15 minutes each day. It can be especially helpful right before bed if you notice your mind is racing.

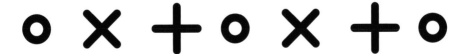

96 Investigate Acupuncture

Acupuncture dates back thousands of years and is rooted in Eastern healing practices. It's based on a concept that all disease, including sleep problems, is the result of an imbalance of subtle energy moving throughout the body. This energy moves along 14 pathways in the body called meridians. Through the ages, practitioners have identified and charted these meridians. Treatment by an acupuncturist involves inserting very fine needles at various points along these meridians to increase, decrease, or balance the energy flow.

In the Western scientific community, there is some skepticism about the use of acupuncture, mainly because there have not been a lot of well-designed, well-controlled studies proving its effectiveness. The National Institutes of Health, however, has stated that there is enough evidence to indicate that acupuncture can be helpful in controlling nausea and certain types of pain. Acupuncture has also been suggested—and in the East, used—as a remedy for insomnia.

It's certainly worth a try, especially for people suffering from chronic pain that affects their ability to get enough restful sleep.

Most people have heard about someone who has been helped by acupuncture but are reluctant to try it themselves because they fear having needles inserted into their body. But the consensus of most people who have used acupuncture is that the procedure causes little or no discomfort, and many swear by the benefits they've received. Side effects from acupuncture are also rare and appear to result mostly from treatment by unqualified practitioners.

If you decide to try acupuncture for your sleep problems, seek out a licensed practitioner, if your state governs this profession, or one certified by the National Certification Commission for Acupuncture and Oriental Medicine (NCCAOM).

97 Get a Massage

Massage is one of several hands-on strategies known collectively as bodywork. And if you've ever had a good, thorough massage, you know the feeling of being "worked over." But you also know how relaxing it can be.

The benefits of massage are many. It is regularly used in sports clinics and rehabilitation centers to loosen or soothe sore, aching muscles. Massage also helps to reduce stress, improve circulation, release tension, lower heart rate and blood pressure, and possibly even strengthen the immune system. These relaxing effects may therefore make massage a helpful aid in restoring restful sleep.

You might want to spring for a massage from a professional. One session may be all it takes to get you hooked. If you do opt for a professional massage, be sure to tell the practitioner if you have any particular illness or injury that they should be aware of, such as arthritis or fibromyalgia.

One of the good things about massage, of course, is that you don't have to visit a professional to capture its benefits. You can ask your partner, friend, or family member for a soothing rubdown. You can also give yourself a mini massage, focusing on the muscle groups that are within reach. Using small, circular movements with your fingers and hands, you can massage your scalp, forehead, face, neck and upper shoulders, lower back, arms, legs, and feet. There are also a variety of massaging devices available in various price ranges that can help extend your reach or provide soothing heat as well as relaxing vibrations.

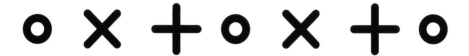

98 Experiment with Aromatherapy

Aromatherapy is the therapeutic use of essential oils to comfort and heal. In aromatherapy, the essential oils are used topically rather than taken internally. The essential oils are said to stimulate an area of the brain known as the limbic system that controls mood and emotion. Solid scientific backing for aromatherapy is lacking, but there's no doubt that many people find it a soothing complement to other self-help measures to ease tension, promote relaxation, and aid in sleep as part of their bedtime preparations.

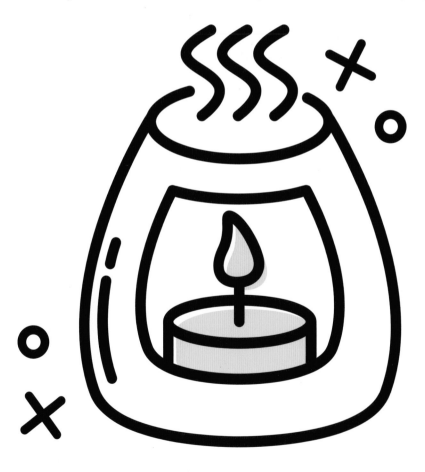

To help restore restful sleep, you can try using essential oils individually or in combination. The essential oils are generally available at health food stores, although these days many drugstores also carry a variety of the oils. The most commonly recommended oil for promoting sleep is lavender, but there are several others that may have a calming effect.

Try adding a few drops of essential oil to warm water for a relaxing bath or footbath, or spritz the oil onto a handkerchief or small pillow. You can also apply a few drops to a heat diffuser near your bed to spread the scent through the room or use a specially made ring that can be placed on the lightbulb of a bedside lamp; the heat of the bulb diffuses the scent.

You might also want to try combining the relaxing benefits of aromatherapy and massage by creating your own scented massage oil. Dilute one to three drops of essential oil per teaspoon of an unscented carrier oil, such as almond or grape-seed oil. (Do not apply undiluted essential oil directly to your skin.) Since some people are more sensitive to the oils than others, start with the smallest amount, and experiment until you find the combination that works best for you.

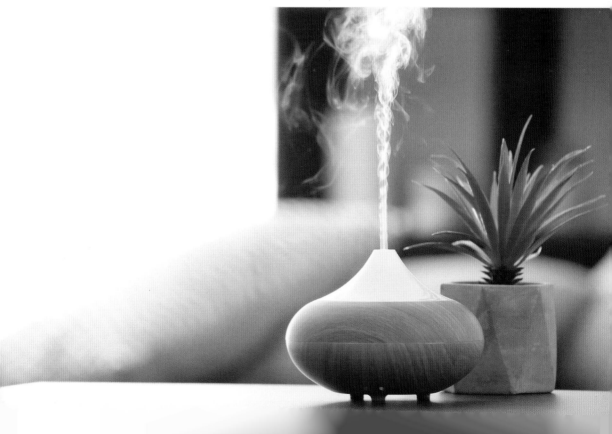

99 Investigate Biofeedback and Self-Hypnosis

Stress can put a major dent in your memory. Toward that end, you may want to try two more techniques: biofeedback and self-hypnosis.

Biofeedback training can help you learn to consciously control certain physical responses to stress. It begins with the use of a simple electronic device that monitors your heart rate, breathing, blood pressure, and/or muscle tension through electrodes that are placed on your skin. These electrodes give "feedback" about what your body is doing under certain conditions. You can then use this feedback to retrain your responses. If you take this route, look for a biofeedback practitioner who is certified by the Biofeedback Certification International Alliance. The option of purchasing inexpensive biofeedback equipment to use on your own is also available.

Self-hypnosis is about obtaining control. A person who is truly hypnotized is in a deep state of relaxation and is fully aware of what is going on around them. For this very reason, self-hypnosis may prove helpful in relieving sleep problems associated with stress. It provides a tool that you can use to induce a deep state of relaxation whenever you want to.

Here's one fairly simple self-hypnosis method. Choose a positive statement that expresses a desire. For instance, "Each breath makes me feel more relaxed." Once you have the statement in mind, lie down and take three slow, deep breaths. Close your eyes and, starting at your head, begin using your affirmation statement on different parts of your body. "Each breath makes my forehead more relaxed." As you breathe, imagine releasing any tension in that part of your body when you exhale. Move to the next part: "Each breath makes my jaw more relaxed." Continue using the same affirmative statement with various parts of your body until you finish with your toes. Continue regular, slow, deep breaths throughout the method.